What Others Are Saying . . .

If you want to know what healing and compassion are all about, read this book, which is a collection of gems drawn from the life of Dr. Anne Brower. It is insights such as these that could transform the profession of medicine. —Larry Dossey, M.D., author of
The Extraordinary Healing Power of Ordinary Things

A deceptively simple book! And a profound statement about the ministry of healing! I Am Not Ready To Die Just Yet *is like a conversation with a wise and trusted friend who knows whereof she speaks. Anne Brower writes compellingly from her experience as priest, physician, and teacher. This is a valuable book for all engaged in pastoral ministry, indeed for all who seek healing for themselves and those they love.*
—Margaret Guenther, Professor Emerita of
General Theological Seminary in New York City
and author of several books on prayer and spirituality

The subtitle to Anne Brower's wonderful book should be, But I Am Ready To Live Fully Now. *From the rich, rare experience as both physician and pastor, Brower presents life as a process of healing emotionally, relationally, and spiritually, as well as physically, so that healing becomes a life of faith. She writes with the clarity of a poet, the spiritual awareness of a pilgrim, the knowledge and experience of a healer, and the compassion of friend as she lays out what she has learned about living fully in the mysterious presence of God. She also writes with the vicissitudes of our humanity, fleshing it out through a variety of stories of real people who become guides for our own pilgrimages. Anne Brower's book is a real blessing. Receive it!*
—Ted Loder, whose latest book is *Loaves,
Fishes and Leftovers: Sharing Life's Deepest Questions*

In this book Anne Brower has shouted out that the healing of the human spirit is an integral part of any effort to cure disease. She does this by numerous examples which also show that spiritual health yields a vibrant life in spite of a body which may be less than perfect.

> —Dr. Howard W. Jones Jr., Professor Emeritus, obstetrics and gynecology at Eastern Virginia Medical School and Johns Hopkins University Medical School. Co-founder of the Jones Institute for Reproductive Medicine.

Whether the end of one's life on earth is near or distant, much comfort will be found in Anne Brower's stories. Her inspiring accounts of friends and patients confronting the ultimate human challenge as well as her own personal journey through a dark valley will touch the reader's heart. This is a treasure of love, compassion, and faith.

> —G. William Whitehurst
> US Congressman (Ret.)

If I were ever to be rector of a congregation again, this book would be required reading for all members of the healing team. Beyond my congregation, it should be required reading for all seminarians and church pastoral care teams. Anne, your theology has caught up with your medical expertise. You are now as experienced a theologian as you are a doctor. The marriage is complete . . . and beautiful.

> —the Reverend James S. Petty,
> Episcopal priest, retired

The Reverend Anne C. Brower, M.D.

I AM NOT READY TO DIE JUST YET

Stories of Healing

Blessings always,
Anne C. Brower

Jan. 2006

R. Brent and Company
Asheville, North Carolina
www.rbrent.com

Published in Asheville, North Carolina
by R. Brent and Company
50 Deerwood Drive
Asheville, NC 28805
828-299-0977
E-mail: robbin@rbrent.com

Editor and Publisher: *Robbin Brent Whittington*
Editors: *Glenn Allen Scott, Libby Riker*
Cover Design: *jb graphics, Asheville, North Carolina*
Radiographic image on cover created by: *Anne Brower, Norfolk, Virginia*
Compositor: *Electronic Publishing Services, Inc., Jonesborough, Tennessee*
Author Photograph: *Vicki Cronis, Virginia Beach, Virginia*

Library of Congress Cataloging-in-Publication Data

Brower, Anne C.
I am not ready to die just yet: stories of healing—1st ed.
      p. cm.
   ISBN-13: 978-0-9678061-7-4
   ISBN-10: 0-9678061-7-8
   1. Health 2. Healing 3. Spirituality
   Title
                              2005936743 LCCN

First Edition

2 4 6 8 10 9 7 5 3 1

Printed in the United States of America

This book is dedicated to:

Karen Janine Davis
who brought forth the divine within me

and to
my husband
Glenn Allen Scott
who gave me the words to express the divine
and who loves me as I love him
through the divine.

Contents

Acknowledgments

I am thankful for the numerous people over the years who have encouraged me to write this book. These are the people who have heard the stories in this book. Thanks specifically go to the Reverend James Petty and the Reverend Margaret Guenther, each of whom always urged me onward. Special thanks to the Canon Reverend Win Lewis who encouraged me to define what healing means and to the Reverend James Hutton who, along with the Canon Reverend Lewis, insisted that I take time away from work to write what they felt would be an important book.

Thanks must be given to the Reverend Dr. Ted Loder who wrote *Guerrillas of Grace* and *My Heart in My Mouth*. His books contain the most beautiful collection of prayers I have ever read. I have used snatches from many of them that fit the wonderful stories in this book. However, the complete prayers, as well as all the others I didn't snatch from, will give the reader of his books unexpected beauty and thought for growth. Our world is a better place because of his prayers.

I would also like to thank Dr. Larry Dossey for mentoring me. I have read every book he has written. I have met him on many occasions at various meetings and we have had wonderful communication between us. I think of him as my guru at whose feet I wish to constantly sit to gather wonderful pearls. How gracious he has been to me. I thank him again.

My deepest and loving thanks go to my husband, Glenn Allen Scott, who edited my book two times, even though he is retired from his profession as editor. It is nice to know that our young marriage was able to survive that phase of this manuscript.

Finally, I would like to thank Robbin Brent Whittington and her staff for turning my manuscript into a beautiful book. Without their ideas, contributions, and editing, this book would still be just a manuscript.

Introduction

This is a book about healing: healing of the whole—mind, body, and spirit.

I am a physician of forty-one years. I have observed, through the radiograph, the intricacies of bone structure and how it changes with time and disease. As I observed these changes, I became acutely aware that the changes in bone, especially the healing of bone, were totally entwined with the healing of the spirit. This seemed to be true with other changes in bone, as well. Therefore, I pursued the path of becoming a priest, so that with the theological understanding of faith and the scientific knowledge of changes in bone, I could speak with more authenticity of the need for healing of the whole—the body, the mind, and the spirit.

Let me demonstrate this healing by illustrating what happens in the fracture of a bone. Mr. Smith breaks the bones in his lower leg—his tibia and fibula—playing soccer. He is treated by aligning the bones as best as possible and surrounding his leg with a plaster cast that goes from above his knee to below his ankle.

Thus encumbered, Mr. Smith is not able to drive a car and so he cannot get to work. He cannot take a shower, unless his leg is sealed inside a garbage bag. He cannot maneuver steps well. He cannot carry anything while walking on his crutches.

The relationship between Mr. Smith and his caregiver (spouse, con-vivant, parent, et al) eventually breaks apart, just as his bones did. Mr. Smith becomes angry because he has lost his independence. His caretaker also becomes angry because his or her routine is disrupted, as he or she provides him with the necessary care. But how dare the caretaker be angry! It's the patient who is hurting. They enter into an unhappy relationship.

Mr. Smith may also break his relationship with God. How often I have seen patients throw down their crutches and exclaim, "Why did God do this to me!" God didn't—but Mr. Smith's anger at God needs to heal as well. All three spheres—body, mind, and spirit—must heal.

The bone begins to heal when osteoclasts (bone-chewing cells) remove the garbage and debris around the fracture. Often a fracture might not be seen immediately on the x-ray, but as the osteoclasts chew away the broken pieces of bone, the fracture becomes visible. This may take a week. Then the osteoblasts (bone-building cells) move in and begin to repair the bone. When the bone is completely reunited by the osteoblasts, it is never the same bone as before the break. The bone may be slightly bent because of inability to obtain perfect alignment. The site of the union is usually much stronger than before it broke.

The two broken relationships must go through the same process. The bad feelings must be openly discussed and cleared away so that, with time, new feelings may take their place. This may create an even stronger relationship between Mr. Smith and his caretaker.

Similarly, the misplaced anger at God must be recognized as such. Knowing or feeling God's presence during his care may bring Mr. Smith to a deeper relationship with God.

In my study of bone changes and healing, I have seen many correlations to spiritual health. Bone is made up of glue—a collagen structure that provides a base—and cement—a mineral structure built upon the glue. When we die, the glue is destroyed by the elements of nature. But nothing can destroy our cement. Just like nothing can destroy our soul. Both live on forever. Should you decide on cremation at the time of death, the ashes that remain are actually pieces of bone. A part of our body will always remain after death, just as our spirit is immortal.

Because bones remain, they are one of the clues that tell us about life in past civilizations. I personally have studied bones more than 5,000 years old in an effort to determine the presence or absence of arthritis. A bone is easier to study than the spirit.

And bones can "die"—osteonecrosis—but still continue to exist if they do not change, respond, or grow. For instance, if the head of the hip dies, it may still serve as the head if it does not respond to the body's attempt to repair it. The same thing happens in your spiritual life—if you do not change, respond, or grow, you become spiritually dead.

As I continued to see the connection of healing at all levels, I studied, observed, and eventually participated in the ancient sacrament of healing—not a sacrament of *curing* but a sacrament of *healing* mind, body, and spirit.

In this book I will tell you what I mean when I talk about healing. In the first two chapters, I define healing and describe the difference between disease, illness, and sickness. In the remaining chapters, I discuss approaches used in healing, with each followed by one to three true stories of healing.

The stories are of people I have known through my studies and practices while becoming a priest and through my career as a physician. They all demonstrate powerfully and inspirationally how people live with, through, and beyond their diseases to a higher health, a higher consciousness, and a deeper relationship with God. Most of the people have since died. I have changed names when necessary of those still living to protect their privacy.

Each story of healing is followed by a prayer, a poem, or a passage of scripture that I feel best describes the person or situation. Each chapter is preceded by an appropriate prayer. The prayers are chosen from many different religions, Christian and non-Christian.

I have many more stories, but I'd rather offer a small selection than go on writing indefinitely. I hope you will be inspired by reading this book as much as I have been moved by the inspirational stories people have related to me; the beauty and power of the prayers, poems, or scripture I have uncovered; and the understanding I have received through many wiser people than I about the healing of the whole—body, mind, and spirit.

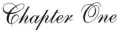

Choosing To Live: Choosing To Heal

Help me to believe in beginnings,
to make a beginning,
to be a beginning,
so that I may not just grow old,
but grow new
each day of this wild, amazing life
you call me to live
with the passion of Jesus Christ.

—Ted Loder[10]

I carry this prayer in my pocket at all times. For I believe that all of us are constantly making beginnings so that we may grow new each day to this wild, amazing life we are called to live with the passion of Jesus Christ. I call living this way *healing.*

Let me define for you disease, cure, and healing. My definitions result from my years of observation as a physician, and as a priest, and from my years of reading as an interested healer. You are welcome to disagree with these definitions.

1

First, disease. My definition starts with what disease is NOT.

Disease is NOT a punishment from God.

Disease is NOT a consequence of sin.

Disease does NOT result from lack of spirituality or lack of effective prayer.

You are NOT guilty, bad, or out of sync with God when you suffer from disease.

Actually, I believe that God created us in *wellness*. If he created us in wellness, then what is disease?

Disease is a process or entity that prevents us from experiencing optimal health. Yet, I would suggest that disease might also be part of the natural order of this universe. After all, if we don't die from a traumatic event, each and every one of us will die from disease.

Look at our universe. Every living thing eventually dies from disease. Trees have tumors, fish have fungi, and my roses have blackspot. We all die. The question is, "What do we die to?"

Nothingness?

Or newness?

I believe we die to newness, to rebirth, to new form, to new life. You and I are witnesses to this every day.

Look at your gardens. Look at the seasons of the year. Look at your own small deaths throughout your life and your beginnings in newness.

My son, who spends his life outdoors, fought the forest fires that ravaged Yellowstone and most of Montana ten or more years ago.

I visited him the following year. I rode with him through charred, black, scarred, decimated forestland. A dispiriting sight.

But the ground was covered with a carpet of new growth—velvet green. My son told me of a specific type of pine that does not release the seed from its cone until the intense heat from a fire reaches it. It appears to me that the natural order of this universe is for death to be followed by rebirth, to be followed by death, to be followed by rebirth, again and again. Disease is a natural part of the process.

Then what is cure?

I define cure as a terminal event. We are cured of disease when we are restored to our original state of being.

You desire to be cured of your disease. As a physician, I wish to cure you of your disease. But, actually, physicians cannot cure most diseases. We can cure pneumonia. But we can only help you to live with diabetes, hypertension, arthritis, cancer, heart disease, alcoholism, and numerous other diseases through medication. We will continue to search for the cure for those diseases we cannot now cure. But ask yourself: After the miracle of a cure, what then? And when there is no cure and we die, we might just have to settle for immortality. Is that so bad?

A *cure* may or may not lead to *healing*. But I believe that in the scheme of the infinite, *cure* is unimportant unless it leads to *healing*.

So what is healing?

Unfortunately, many of us associate healing with disease. As a younger physician, I believed my job was to *heal* my patients of their physical or mental afflictions. I confused *cure* with *healing*.

Through experience, observation, reading, and study, I arrived at a much more expansive definition of healing.

I believe healing is a way of life that leads towards total communion—oneness—with God. Nothing more, nothing less.

Healing is a lifelong process involving change, growth, progress, regress, and beginnings that help us to grow new.

Healing demands of us love and surrender.

Healing is NOT limited to disease. Healing is our life.

Healing is living with, through, and beyond brokenness—brokenness from disease, divorce, loss or change of job, relocation, loss of friend or family, loss of rector . . . .

Healing is moving out of the box we may be stuck in.

Healing is always moving toward a closer union with God.

I believe that Jesus' life is a story of healing.

Yes, he cured. He enabled the blind to see, the deaf to hear, the withered hand to become whole, the paralytic to walk, and the woman's blood to stop flowing. But each time he cured, he did so to bring healing to humankind—to reveal to us the kingdom of God, to raise us to a higher health, to make known to us the divine within each of us.

I believe that he would not have cured if he could have taught us about God in any other way. Had his mission been to cure disease, he would have cured everyone, not just a few.

Countless avenues are available to lead us to this healing way of life: meditation, prayer, music, art, gardening, dance, anything creative. We are co-creators with God.

One avenue is the healing rite, an ancient holy sacrament of the church. One presents oneself to God for prayer and laying on of hands. This rite leads to a deeper communion with God. Nothing less, nothing more. (See chapter 6.)

Here is a story I learned from another physician, Larry Dossey.

A man dying of lung cancer was in the hospital for his last week of life.

He was not a religious man. He had never read the Bible, he had never been to church, he had never opened a prayer book.

Nonetheless, the dying man asked to see a chaplain a few days before he died. He told the chaplain that during his waking hours for the past three weeks he had been praying incessantly. He then asked the chaplain to please pray with him and lay hands upon him—*the healing rite.*

"What are you praying for?" the chaplain asked.

The man laughed.

"I'm not praying for anything. I know I'm almost dead. My wife is dead. I have no children. I've finished my job. Nothing is left in this world for me. There really is nothing for me to pray for."

"Then why are you praying?" asked the chaplain.

"Because," the dying man replied, "it helps me to know that I am not alone."

That's what *healing* is all about—knowing you are with God.

Elizabeth: Not Ready to Die Just Yet

Elizabeth was a pillar of the community and of the church to which she had belonged since childhood. Everybody knew her. One of the many things she did was run a very busy gift shop for the church. I remember when Beanie Babies were the thing to have. She was the first in town to stock them. She always had the very newest ones. She bought unique merchandise for the shop and then persuaded you that you needed this or that item for yourself or as a gift. She had a wonderful sense of humor and an infectious laugh. Everyone liked to visit the shop just to talk with her.

Elizabeth awakened one morning with chest pain. She saw her internist, who immediately referred her to a cardiologist. In less than twelve hours, she was in the cardiac lab having a cardiac catheterization. Unfortunately, as the catheter traversed the artery towards the heart, it knocked a piece of plaque off the wall of her artery. The piece of plaque lodged in her brain, which produced a massive stroke that paralyzed her right side.

She was immediately taken to radiology where the doctors attempted to dissolve the offending piece of plaque, but the piece was not within reach. Combined with all the medication she received during the various procedures, the stroke left her temporarily comatose. The next day, she regained her cognitive powers but none of the motor skills of her right arm and right leg.

Elizabeth's mother had suffered a stroke and, after three years of intensive care provided by Elizabeth, died. This experience soured Elizabeth on living as a stroke victim. She had signed a living will and had carefully instructed her family that if she ever suffered a disabling stroke she was to be allowed to die. While she was briefly comatose, Elizabeth's family and doctors honored her explicit instructions that she be given no food and no liquids, either by mouth or intravenously.

Elizabeth's emergence from her coma posed a moral dilemma for some. Although Elizabeth had regained her cognitive powers, her physicians and family—in accord with the instructions in her living will—continued to give her nothing by mouth or intravenously.

The rector of her church visited her every day. His Sunday sermon three days after Elizabeth's hospitalization praised her glorious presence in the church and all but announced her death.

The associate rector was enraged that Elizabeth was being deprived of sustenance. He believed that as long as Elizabeth's mind was competent, her life should be sustained.

The dilemma divided her friends. Some were outraged that nothing was being done to save her from dying; others were praising her courage for choosing to die.

The doctors continued to honor her living will and her family's wishes. Her son had been in a serious motorcycle accident and was severely handicapped. He was stuck in a box with his "illness." He was very angry and bitter that he had survived the crash.

Ironically, it was his mother's care that had kept him alive. He strongly hoped to spare his mother a fate similar to his. But the nurses, troubled by starving to death a stroke victim with cognitive abilities, called the ethics committee of the hospital for help.

Many people visited Elizabeth in the hospital. All were shocked by the change in her appearance. Paralyzed by the stroke and lacking food and liquid, her bright buoyant spirit had disappeared. She wasn't the Elizabeth they had known before her stroke. This made most of her visitors, including the rector, very uncomfortable. Most didn't talk *with* Elizabeth; they talked *at* her.

They wished her well.

They prayed for her.

But no one asked Elizabeth what she wanted.

No one listened to her.

Elizabeth and I were not close friends, but we had rapport. Because I was known in the church as a physician and lay person with a passion for healing, several of her friends asked me to visit her. What was happening to Elizabeth made no sense to them. "Elizabeth can carry on a rational conversation," the rector told me, "but she has no ability to discern and often displays inappropriate emotions. She is crying a great deal. I don't believe that her crying is appropriate."

The rector's report made no sense to me, so I agreed to see her. I arrived in her hospital room just a few hours before the family was coming to take her home to die.

When I entered her room, Elizabeth appeared to be dozing.

I said, gently, "Elizabeth, it's me, Anne, from the church."

She was instantly alert.

"Oh, I'm so glad you came to see me!"

I was surprised and pleased by her obvious delight. Her response suggested that she had been hoping I would come.

I noted that the stroke had not affected the movement of her facial muscles; nor had it affected her speech.

I pulled up a chair and held her right hand. A lengthy silence ensued while she struggled with what she wanted to say. She broke the silence.

"I need to ask you a question—may I?"

"Of course."

"They are going to have a big meeting this afternoon—the doctors, my family, my rector, and others. They are trying to decide whether to put a feeding tube in me or not. They say I will starve to death without a feeding tube."

Tears filled her eyes.

"Well," I said, "if you are unable to swallow, then you will starve to death without the feeding tube."

"But I *can* swallow," she said. "The nurses sneak me yogurt at night when no one else is around."

I was astonished, but said nothing. I continued to hold her hand and remained calm.

Another long silence.

Suddenly she spoke. "Well, I don't think that I am ready to die just yet."

More tears filled her eyes.

"Perhaps it's not time for you to die yet, Elizabeth. Perhaps God wants a few days or more for you right now."

"Well," she responded, "I have this living will that the family has invoked."

To which I responded, "Yes, I understand that. But as long as you are competent mentally, which you are, your living will need not be in effect, if you choose for it not to be."

"The doctors tell me that I will never recover from this stroke—that I will always be like this."

Now I'm angry. I'm angry that her physicians told her that she wouldn't recover. They had no right to say that. It was much too early in the course of her stroke to know the outcome. Who were they? God?

"No one right now," I said vehemently, "can possibly know what will happen to you. You may get worse, you may get better, or you may stay the same. It's too early to know. No one has the right to tell you otherwise. It's really between you and God."

"Well," Elizabeth said, "I wish I could know whether I'll get better or not."

"Of course you do!" I said. "But trust that God is with you and will help provide those answers as you need them."

Yet another long silence.

"I want to do what is right for my family." She was now crying more.

"And they want to do what is right for you," I said. "So you need to decide what is right for *you*."

We spoke briefly of other things and then I excused myself, for she was very tired, and very weak, both from the stroke and the lack of nourishment.

She found her voice at the big meeting that afternoon.

"I don't wish to die yet!" Elizabeth announced.

She was immediately transferred to the rehabilitation ward.

I visited her the next morning. She was sitting up, eating an enormous breakfast, and ready to learn how to use her disabled arm and leg. She looked so happy.

Her embittered son entered the room. Elizabeth introduced me as the woman who had saved her life.

"And just what did you tell my mother?" he asked angrily.

I dodged the bullet by replying, "I didn't tell her anything. I think she just listened to God."

Elizabeth beamed from ear to ear.

She never regained full function of her right side. She was wheelchair-bound. But she wrote notes to many people with her right hand. She lived another five years, before another stroke ended her life.

Those five years for Elizabeth were not at all like the unhappy years she remembered her mother enduring after her stroke. Elizabeth's five years were glorious, even though she had to exert herself heroically to restore limited function to her right side and needed assistance from her husband, daughter, and nurses.

During those five years, she traveled to trade shows with others to purchase items for the gift shop. She helped to run the gift shop, as she had in the past. She visited with friends. She watched her grandchildren grow. She and her devoted husband celebrated their fiftieth wedding anniversary in exquisite style with a flood of family and friends.

Elizabeth was loved.

Elizabeth was able to say her goodbyes.

Each day of those five years was a gift from God.

Elizabeth knew that and rejoiced.

Heaven's not a rest;
No! but to battle with new zest,
Untired, with warrior joy,
The sharp keen spirit to employ
On life's new enterprise,
It's the surprise
Of keen delighted mind
That wakes, to find
Old fetters gone,
Strong shining immortality put on.

—Anonymous[3]

Dorothy and Friends:
Riding Beyond Their Afflictions

For years I have vacationed at a ranch southwest of Tucson, twenty miles north of the Mexican border. I am continually awed by the courage and bravery manifested by many of the guests. They inspire me.

Many live in New England or the northern-tier states and come to the ranch in winter to escape the cold back home. And they come to ride.

Guests who come to the ranch once tend to return year after year. Many have come for thirty or more years, stopping only when they are too ill or when they die. The ranch provides safe space to nourish one's self in solitude and yet expand one's horizons through a delightful community at mealtime and on group rides. The ranch staff honors the elderly and handicapped by making every effort to ensure that their vacation is as fulfilling for them as it is for other guests. The guests become friends.

Dorothy

Dorothy was ninety-four years old when she vacationed for the last time at the ranch. She would still ride every day. And on the days when we could choose an all-day ride, she would choose that ride. She dismounted her horse for lunch, used the "outdoor" facilities more easily than I, who was fifty-four at the time, and remounted her horse limberly.

Back in her cabin at day's end, Dorothy tidied herself and hosted a cocktail hour for a group of us. She played bridge after dinner, her mind keener than most of the other minds at the bridge table. Some evenings, after a guitarist performed, she urged the guitarist to play the "oldies but goodies" for us all to sing while she danced.

Dorothy did not know that that vacation was to be her final one. She returned to her home in Michigan to host a dinner for the local symphony. The dinner was catered. But she made the dessert, swans, using a recipe she discovered at the ranch. The swans were puff pastry shells filled with whipped cream, each with an extra piece of pastry twisted to make a swan's neck. It took great patience and dexterity to make one.

She died six months later.

Jack

Jack had been a longtime annual vacationer at the ranch when a stroke paralyzed the right side of his body. Several years later, his daughter brought him back to the ranch. He mounted a horse every day. A mounted wrangler led Jack's horse by a rope. A guest rider usually followed Jack. Having no sensation on the right side of his body, Jack tended to lean to the left. When he came close to falling off, either the wrangler or the rider behind would tell Jack to straighten up. He straightened up by using his left hand on the saddle horn to pull himself to the right.

He always asked, "Am I straight enough?"

When he was, he could ride for another thirty minutes.

George

George had had two total-knee replacements, but on a horse, he rode better than he walked. It took the wranglers' time and patience helping him mount the horse, but they never showed any sign of this being an inconvenience.

Penny

Penny lived with severe emphysema—so severe that she needed to ride in a golf cart from her cabin to the main dining room, a distance of one hundred feet. She still rode her horse every day and chose an all-day ride when all-day rides were scheduled. She did not even take an oxygen tank with her when she rode.

She, I, and other guests always had spirited and deep conversations over dinner. She never talked about her disease.

Nan

At age seventy-nine, Nan was struck by an automobile while she was walking. The collision caused fractures of her right shoulder, right leg, three cervical vertebrae, and the base of her skull. She was in the hospital for nine weeks, during which time she underwent three operations. Nan remembered nothing of the first six weeks. Her cervical spine was fused. She had hardware in her shoulder and in her lower right leg. She was eighty-one when she returned to the ranch. She had not ridden a horse for three years. On her first ride, she rode for ninety minutes. Thinking she had overdone it, she rode for sixty minutes the next time and felt better.

Ruth

Ruth, who was in her sixties, had ridden horses since her childhood. She was a very heavy woman with a great spirit.

Three years before, she had a total hip replacement. The hip replacement became infected twice and was replaced each time. She lost length in her leg. While undergoing exercises to lengthen the leg, she broke her femur. She walked like the Hunchback of Notre Dame, with crutches to support her every step. She returned to the ranch for the first time three years after her initial surgery. Mounting the horse required the assistance of four wranglers in addition to her own strenuous efforts. But once in the saddle, she rode like she always had before.

Sue

Sue, another longtime annual ranch guest, lost her eyesight. The loss occurred slowly over several years. Totally blind, she still rode her horse with the rest of the guests. The rider in front of Sue alerted her to duck her head when approaching low-hanging tree branches, to guide her horse to the right to avoid thorny cactuses, and to not let her horse drink while crossing a stream. The rider in front was Sue's eyes.

What great perseverance these riders showed. What great determination to return to the life they enjoyed so much in their younger years. What courage they had to try again, though severely hindered by their traumas or their diseases. They rode with their wounds, but also beyond their wounds.

They were not ready to die just yet.

A COWBOY'S PRAYER

O Lord, I've never run where churches grow,
I've always loved Creation better as it stood
That day you finished it, so long ago,
And looked upon your work, and found it good.

Let me be easy on the man that's down
And make me square and generous with all;
I'm careless sometimes, Lord, when I'm in town,
But never let them call me mean or small.

—Elliot Perkins[3]

Ruby: God's Next Assignment

I met Ruby near the end of her life. The retirement-home chaplain asked me to call on Ruby because she had "gone through so much." At that time, Ruby resided in the independent-living section of the retirement complex.

Ruby did not greet me at the door of her apartment; she called through the door, inviting me in.

I opened the door. Ruby was seated in a reclining chair, watching the television screen directly before her. Beside her was a table on wheels containing all of her necessities: Kleenex, medications, water, snacks, books. She had arranged a compact living area within her moderate-size living room.

Ruby was short and thin. Her gray hair was cropped very short and the lenses in her glasses were very thick.

She had been napping, but my presence brought her to life. As we conversed, she became vivacious, excited, often sitting straight up and swinging her legs off the recliner.

She coughed frequently and attempted often to clear her throat. Talking was extremely difficult for her, but she didn't want to stop. She had difficulty breathing. She said she had learned of my work at the retirement home and had very much wanted to speak with me.

Her story is heartrending.

About a year and a half before we met, she had attended a play with a group from the retirement home. The play, Neil Simon's "The Odd Couple," is about the tensions between two divorced males sharing an apartment to save money. The version of the play seen by Ruby replaced the lead characters with two divorced women.

Ruby laughed so hard that she suddenly developed severe pain in her chest.

Because the pain persisted, her chest was x-rayed. The x-ray revealed that she had broken a rib while laughing so hard. Worse, the x-ray also showed a shadow the size of a pea in her right lung.

Ruby's physician chose to monitor the shadow with monthly chest x-rays for six months. By then, the pea had grown to the size of a quarter. Only then was the lesion biopsied. Ruby was diagnosed with lung cancer.

Ruby was offered a choice. She could undergo the normal protocol of chemotherapy, which probably would allow her to live a year to a year and a half longer. The other choice was an experimental protocol using massive doses of radiation and chemotherapy within a very brief period.

Ruby's doctors thought the second regimen might produce a longer remission of her cancer or, possibly, a total cure.

Ruby chose the short course of massive radiation and chemotherapy, hoping to extend her life and perhaps be cured.

The treatment proved to be worse than the disease. Ruby was extremely sick throughout the therapy. She was confined to bed and totally dependent upon family and friends to take care of her.

"The chemotherapy wasn't the bad one," Ruby told me many months after her treatment was complete. "It was the radiation. I felt scorched; I felt like I was charcoal inside. I felt burned to death."

She was speaking the truth, although she had no way of knowing how much damage the radiation had inflicted upon her chest. Radiation had burned the skin on her chest severely. The skin was now totally scarred.

"I would never go through that again," she told me. "I really would rather die. But if God wants me to do some more here on Earth, the treatment will work. If he doesn't, the treatment won't work. It's okay either way."

"Are you afraid of dying?" I asked.

"No. Not at all," she replied. "I just thought I'd like to live a few more years, if possible. You know, this really has been the best of years and the worst of years."

Following her treatment and a short rest, Ruby and her sisters traveled together to Budapest, Vienna, Prague, and throughout much of Germany, ending up at Oberammagau, to see the Passion Play—the play was the highlight of her life. For years and years, she had wished to see the Passion Play. Telling me about it, she re-experienced every moment. With great excitement, she described all the images and stories. In a sense, she had lived for that one day.

"This trip must have required a lot of energy," I said. "How did you manage?"

"Oh, I took naps. And sometimes I wouldn't go with my sisters. I paced myself but saw everything I ever wanted to see." The trip lasted three weeks.

A month after her return home, her children threw a birthday party celebrating her eighty years of life.

"I wouldn't have missed that for the world," Ruby told me.

Ruby went for a CAT scan upon her return to determine the presence or absence of her cancer. The result was indeterminate because she had "too much congestion in her lung." (The "congestion" actually was death of lung tissue from the radiation.) Another CAT scan three months later was also indeterminate.

I saw Ruby several times after that visit. Her physical health was deteriorating rapidly. But she was mentally sharp and remarkably cheerful and optimistic. Eventually she required oxygen around the clock.

Before she was tied to an oxygen tank, she still visited her children and grandchildren, always enjoying her times with them and excited when telling me about her visits.

The last time I saw Ruby, she had been moved to the nursing-home section of the retirement home. The lung cancer had metastasized to her brain. A small dose of radiation had been administered to her brain to shrink the metastatic lesions. She had lost her hair and was wearing a colorful bandanna around her head. She was in the physical-therapy room, where she basically was visiting the other patients there, "helping them to keep their spirits up."

"Maybe this is the work God has kept me alive to do," Ruby said.

She died not long afterwards, with, I was told, a smile on her face.

So, God, this is what I ask,
    that you would pull off in me
        this one miracle quick enough
            to finish in my short remaining years.
Perhaps you've begun, I hope,
    by giving me pause to rest in this prayer,
        which is to rest in you.
            Thank you. Amen.

—Ted Loder[11]

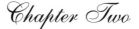

Finding Wholeness: Disease vs Illness and Sickness

Let us be filled with the presence of the great compassion towards ourselves and towards all living beings.

—A New Zealand Prayer Book (163)[13]

hose who had known Jesus before his crucifixion usually did not immediately recognize Jesus after his resurrection. Why?

Basically, one of two things occurred that eventually made people aware of his presence. Either he was sharing supper or he appeared with the wounds that he received on the cross—the nail holes in his hands, the nail holes through his feet, and the spear wound in his side. He was identified by his wounds.

While he lived, Jesus shared meals with the marginal men and women of society. He also cured—usually one person at a time—the lame, the blind, the deaf, the paralytic, the hemorrhaging woman, the man with the withered arm, the lepers. He did this to teach the crowds about the kingdom of God, and that God was present not only around them, but also within each one of them.

Why was Jesus resurrected with his crucifixion wounds? Why didn't he appear whole or healed?

I believe he did appear whole (healed) through his still-visible wounds.

I believe he was telling us that his horrible wounds were unimportant to his wholeness. The wounds did not affect him.

I believe Jesus was teaching us how to live. For all of us will forever have our own wounds—disease, loss, abuse, depression—but can we, like Christ, not only live *with* them, but also *through* and *beyond* them?

I believe that is what he asks us to do. Since brokenness at some point in our lives is inevitable—it is the human condition—Jesus challenges us to live beyond our brokenness to a higher health, a higher consciousness.

Disease is one of the foremost causes of brokenness. How can we live beyond our disease? Understanding the difference between disease, illness, and sickness may be helpful.

Disease is inevitable.

Illness and sickness are not.

Medical anthropologist Allan Young separates disease into three components: disease, illness, and sickness.[18] Brokenness of any kind can be separated into the same three components.

Young defines disease as "the organic pathologies and abnormalities" that attack us. Diabetes, rheumatoid arthritis, and cancer are among many of the diseases that afflict human beings. Divorce is one example of an event, rather than a disease, that leads to brokenness.

"Illness," Young writes, "is how the disease or brokenness is brought into the individual consciousness." Whether "disease" becomes "illness" is determined by how the person with a disease perceives and responds to the disease. "Disease" is transformed into "illness" when one thinks or says, "I am suffering from diabetes [arthritis, cancer, or other disease]," instead of "I have diabetes [arthritis, cancer, or other disease], but I can still appreciate each moment of every day."

Young defines "sickness as the process through which worrisome behavioral and biological signs are given socially recognizable meanings." Society creates sickness by avoiding, detaching, or isolating itself from the one who has the disease. A person with disease may be able to function competently in society, but society doesn't want to be involved or associated with that diseased person. Society's reaction to people with AIDS illustrates the most obvious modern-day example of how "disease" becomes "sickness." People with AIDS, cancer, or SARS are called "victims." The word "victim" in itself exemplifies sickness.

"Illness" personalizes disease. "Sickness" socializes both disease and illness. Sickness can produce illness and vice versa; but disease need not coexist with illness and sickness.

We may be able to do little to change disease, but we can try hard to prevent illness and sickness. Jesus couldn't stop his crucifixion. But he transformed his "disease" not into "illness" but into glorious resurrection. He stopped all "sickness" three days after his crucifixion by appearing whole while still bearing his wounds—the signs of his "disease."

Stories of people living with disease, yet beyond illness and sickness, are presented throughout this book. An artist whose disease, rheumatoid arthritis, disabled her so she couldn't paint with her right hand did not succumb to "illness"—she learned to paint with her left hand. Society let go of her "sickness" when she let go of her "illness." (See Harriet's story.)

We already read about Elizabeth, who had a paralyzing stroke and became "ill" for a few days after telling herself that she should not burden her family by continuing to live. Her family and doctors transformed her illness into sickness for a few days as they honored her living will. But within a week she dismissed her illness and her sickness as she regained her desire to live and demanded to be rehabilitated. (See Elizabeth's story.)

I am a breast-cancer survivor. Breast cancer was my disease. I had just moved to a new job in a city where I had never lived before. I had no community. I was lonely and depressed. I had become "ill."

A few friends made me "sick" by saying, "Oh, Anne, you always travel with your glass half empty instead of half full" and, "You're going to have to change your lifestyle after you get through this, for obviously you brought this cancer on yourself by living too fast." These were but two dismissive and depreciative comments made about my situation. (See Anne's story, part one.)

By society's standards, I was sick. Months passed before I got beyond my illness and my sickness. I found new friends. One friend made me feel whole again through massage and spiritual direction. Other friends, through caring, drove away my depression. My new friends banished my "sickness" by taking away my "illness." (See Anne's story, part two.)

Now I am whole, but still with the scars from my cancer. Healing has occurred, the healing that Jesus modeled for all of us.

Jesus expressed his own "illness" when he cried out, "My God, my God, why have you forsaken me?"

He endured his own "sickness" when his disciples slept instead of keeping watch while he prayed in Gethsemane, betrayed him, and then deserted him.

Then he returned to all of us, healed and whole, yet with his wounds—his "disease"—telling us that all is well with him, including his wounds.

Mattie: Healing Wings

Mattie is eighty-nine years old. When I first met her several years ago, she was coming into the hallway of the assisted-living unit from the outside, all bundled up for winter, walking with the aid of a bright red walker with wheels.

A bright red basket on the walker held two empty gallon jugs for water, a scrub brush, and a bag of birdseed. She was quite intent on where she was going and did not see me.

I spoke.

She smiled and invited me into her room for a chat.

Mattie suffers with fibrosis of her lungs—which makes it difficult for her to breathe—and liver failure. Both of these problems are known unwelcome side effects of the drug she had been treated with for too long.

Mattie took off her coat with difficulty, pushed her cart aside, and, puffing and coughing, sat down in her favorite chair.

But her eyes were bright and alive and she was ready to talk.

"You know my liver is so big I told them they could give some of it to someone else. But I guess it's too sick."

"Do you feel sick?" I asked.

"Not to worry," she replied, "I'm tough as nails."

I was curious about the contents of her walker basket. So she told me that she had always wanted a birdbath just outside her window. She asked her daughter to give her one for Christmas, but her daughter dismissed her request; a birdbath, her daughter said, would be too difficult for Mattie to take care of.

So Mattie bought one herself. In a catalog, she found a birdbath that was "beautiful—black, sleek, and smooth. And the inside was painted gold."

When the birdbath arrived, she found a maintenance man at the retirement home to help her put it up. She told me all this with great pride.

But the birdbath rusted.

"Can you imagine that?" she asked. "How could such a beautiful thing rust? Well, I had spent one hundred dollars for it, but the catalog guaranteed total satisfaction or your money back. So I got help wrapping it up and sent it back. Got my money back."

Her daughter then understood how serious Mattie was about acquiring a birdbath and bought her one with a stone pedestal and plastic top—a top that Mattie could lift off to dump the water. So every morning, Mattie fills her stroller basket with two gallons of water, the scrub brush, and the birdseed. At the birdbath, she scrubs the plastic top, lifts the top, dumps the dirty water, fills the top with fresh water, and then sprinkles some seed around the pedestal so the birds will come.

Mattie takes the entire morning doing these things. Then she watches the birds every afternoon from her chair. The birds' antics are such a delight for her.

"It keeps me going," she says, "and I enjoy the birds so much."

During one of my visits, Mattie seemed quite tired. She had been to an ophthalmologist who wanted to remove a cataract from her eye immediately. She had refused, because the ophthalmologist didn't know about her lung or liver diseases.

She also had recently developed superficial infections on her legs. The nurses were wrapping her legs twice a day with antibiotic-coated gauze wraps, and this therapy seemed to be tiring her.

"I might die tomorrow of these infections," she said.

I asked her if she really believed that.

"No," she said. "But my cataract certainly doesn't need to be removed right now. My mortality is right here with me, so why waste time on something that isn't harming me?"

On another visit I asked what she was doing for Thanksgiving. She led me over to her piled-up kitchen counter and pulled out a box of beautifully decorated stationery, many decorated with birds. She showed me one card on which she had written her own beautiful faith-filled poem. She had placed quotations taken from a day-by-day calendar around her poem and heart stickers above her signed name.

"This is what I do for Thanksgiving. I send these to all those with whom I might have shared Thanksgiving. I get lots of invitations for Thanksgiving, but I don't think I should take my cough, my infected legs, and my incontinence into someone else's house. These cards would mean so much more than my unhealthy presence." I didn't tell her, but I disagreed with her decision to turn down invitations. Because, despite her unhealthy body, she had so much spirit and love to share.

Mattie truly is a tough person—demanding and commanding. I am sure these qualities help her to live beyond her disease.

But she is also very tender and loving—demonstrated by the care she gives the birds and the cards she sends. Mattie is still needed here in God's earthly creation.

I haven't seen Mattie for more than a year now. But this Christmas I received one of her wonderful cards with ten dollars enclosed for me to use in my work. I intend to use it well.

For making me a woman
in what still so often
seems a man's world,
I thank you.
Because you taught me by example
that power is your gift,
and not my possession.

For giving me a body
though it sometimes fails me
and is not all I wish it was
or rather, a good deal more
than I wish it was,
I thank you.
Because you taught me
that I am much more
than my body
and yet my body is
your holy temple.

For calling me to be
more than I believe I can be,
and less
than I sometimes pretend I am,
I thank you.
Because you taught me
that being is more than doing,
that who I am
and whose I am
are more important than
what I do
or what I have.

For all that you are
Creator,
Redeemer,
Sanctifier,
Great "I Am,"
I bless you
as you have so greatly blessed me.

—Ms. Marty Conner[6]

Sylvia: A Life of Many Beginnings

Sylvia and I were very close friends.

She came late into my life; our years together were brief. She was twenty years older than I was.

I knew Sylvia first as the consultant to the board creating the Pastoral Care, Counseling, and Education Center at St. Columba's Episcopal Church in Washington, D.C. She saw qualities in me that led her to make me president of the board. I looked to her for guidance at all times, and we became friends.

Sylvia developed and ran the nursery school at St. Columba's. It was then, and still is, the most prestigious nursery school in D.C.

Her husband was an oceanographer. She and her husband had two children before he joined the armed forces in World War II and three more following the war. She explained, "I had two families with the same man."

She worked all the time as head of the St. Columba's nursery school and loved every minute, and the children loved her. She retired reluctantly, when her husband retired from his oceanographer's job. She retired to be free to travel around the world with him.

But they didn't get to travel together. Sylvia's husband died unexpectedly from a massive stroke about one month after their retirements. Sylvia couldn't do much for about a year because of her deep grief over her husband's death.

But then she moved on. She could not return to the school, for she had chosen her replacement. She became a consultant to church search committees seeking the right rectors to serve their parishes.

She was so good at assisting search committees that she became everyone's first choice as a consultant. She also consulted with vestries disenchanted with their clergy.

She traveled with me to out-of-town medical meetings, visiting places she had never been before.

On one of our trips, we traveled to Albuquerque, where she had gone to high school and lived as a new bride. She was so excited about returning "home" for a visit. We extended this trip to Santa Fe, New Mexico.

In Santa Fe, I learned just how small the world is and how connected we all are. Sylvia accompanied me to visit Eleanor, a friend of my mother's, whose husband had just recently died.

Eleanor's eyes were very blue and her hair was pure white. For most of her adult years, she had taught very young Navajo Indian children how to brush their teeth and comb their hair.

Sylvia's eyes were also very blue and her hair pure white and, of course, she had for many years taught three- and four-year-olds.

The story is too long to tell here, but during that evening in Santa Fe Sylvia and Eleanor discovered that they shared the same grandmother. Each had spent separate summers at their grandmother's house, so they had never known each other.

Sylvia's mother had moved to a ranch in Colorado Springs subsequently acquired by the United States Air Force Academy. Eleanor's mother had moved to Pasadena, California. Sylvia and Eleanor, both in their seventies, had much to tell each other about their families and themselves. An evening that started out to be short became very long and filled with exciting discoveries.

Sylvia was always a pioneer. As a child in Colorado, she trapped beavers and stripped them of their pelts. She took the pelts to the post office on the way to school and collected twenty-five cents per pelt on her way back home.

Sylvia met her husband in Colorado when she was fifteen and married him against everyone's wishes.

Her husband was a geologist at that time. She followed him to Albuquerque where he had a job. In those days you could not attend high school if you were married. But that didn't deter Sylvia. She marched into the principal's office the first day and demanded, "You aren't going to keep me from an education I should have, are you?" The principal didn't. He admitted Sylvia, who then completed her secondary-school education. But her husband was not allowed to attend her senior prom.

Sylvia introduced me to Dr. Larry Dossey. She had read an advertisement in *The Washington Post* newspaper promoting Dossey's book *Healing Words.*[4] She had not read the book, but she knew intuitively that the book was meant for me.

"I am sure this will help you with your work," Sylvia said.

She was exactly right. Reading *Healing Words* changed my life.

About five years before Sylvia died, she underwent a total hip replacement for osteonecrosis (death of the bone). She healed swiftly from the surgery.

You couldn't keep Sylvia down. Her physician warned her that placing her leg in a certain position might dislocate her hip. Since she experienced no postoperative pain, she repeatedly forgot to keep her leg out of the dangerous position.

I thought she was going to kill me each time I pointed out that her leg was wrongly positioned. One time she really blew up at me when I asked her to reposition her leg safely. But she was actually mad at herself, angry that her mobility was restricted during this healing period. Especially because she felt so well.

On the day I arrived in D.C. to bury my mother, who had died unexpectedly, Sylvia told me she herself had been very short of breath and had some fluid removed from her lung.

The fluid contained malignant cells. Three days later, while on her way to have a mammogram to determine the primary site of the cancer, she suffered a transient ischemic episode (a short-lived stroke). An ambulance took her to the emergency room, where a CAT scan revealed two metastatic lesions in her brain—one was the size of an orange.

How had she lived such a normal life with so much disease? I obtained her chest x-ray from the time of her hip surgery five years before. The x-ray showed a dime-size lesion, with tentacles.

There was her cancer. But her doctors had missed it. Her new doctors had not seen it this time either, because the fluid in her lung had obscured it.

I said nothing to Sylvia or her doctors, because the prognosis for a person with lung cancer that had metastasized to this extent was six months at best.

I believe that Sylvia already knew, without anyone telling her, that she would die soon.

She was treated with radiation to her brain in an effort to shrink the size of the large metastatic lesion and thus protect her quality of life. But her quality of life began to deteriorate with each radiation treatment. She said she felt okay, but I found her often confused and disoriented.

I returned to Norfolk, keeping in touch with Sylvia by telephone. I drove back to Washington, D.C. a month later to see her, expecting that she would greet me at her front door with her winning smile and warm hugs and that we would later eat the dinner she had prepared for us. She had told me that just such a welcome awaited me when we had spoken on the telephone the day before.

But the promised welcome was not to be. Instead, I found Sylvia in bed. She welcomed me from her bed with her smile, saying, "I just didn't feel like getting up today."

I was shocked by her appearance and her apparent unawareness of how greatly her health had deteriorated.

I fixed us some food and fed her as she lay in bed. After we had eaten, I lay on the floor next to her bed and we listened to music that she loved.

She couldn't see me on the floor, which allowed me to cry very softly. She never knew the immense sadness I felt.

I still cry when remembering that time.

I telephoned one of her sons the next morning. None of her children had understood just how very sick she was.

Family members came immediately from all over—including Hawaii. They had a good week with Sylvia before she slipped into a coma. She remained in a coma for three days and then died peacefully.

As a physician for nearly four decades, I've learned—much to my amazement—that the bodies of some people are able to control a disease for lengthy periods before the disease becomes manifest.

Most of us will die from one of seven causes—cancer, infection, arteriosclerosis of the arteries to the heart, hypertension, diabetes, senile dementia, or obesity.[14] Autopsies reveal that people who have died from one of these causes may harbor one or several other diseases that have not become manifest to the deceased before death.

Sylvia lived as a well person with extensive disease attacking her body for five years. Neither she nor her physicians had detected the cancer until her life had nearly ended. I'm glad she didn't know that she had lung cancer for five years.

Why?

Had the lesion been detected earlier during those five years, she would have had it surgically removed and then gone through the tough ordeal of chemotherapy—only to die about when she did die.

As it was, she lived fully and enthusiastically for five years, unaware of the disease that had attacked her. She had a quality five years. She was ill very briefly before succumbing to her cancer.

Sylvia was such a pioneer throughout her life, making new beginnings in every phase of her life, and doing them well. I think and speak of her often; she remains a presence in my life. She was a blessing to so many people.

Do not stand at my grave and weep;
I am not there. I do not sleep.
I am a thousand winds that blow;
I am the diamond glints on snow.
I am the sunlight on ripened grain;
I am the gentle autumn rain.
When you awaken in the morning's hush,
I am the swift uplifting rush
Of quiet birds in circled flight.
I am the soft stars that shine at night.
Do not stand at my grave and cry,
I am not there; I did not die.

—Navajo burial prayer[3]

Harriet: "I'm a Survivor"

I first met Harriet early during my journey toward priesthood. All people seeking entrance into seminary must fulfill several requirements of the ordination exploration process, a process established for me by the Episcopal Diocese of Southern Virginia. One requirement was working in a local church as a student-clergyperson for four months. I was assigned to work with the clergy of St. Mark's Episcopal Church in Hampton, Virginia. Harriet was a member of the committee appointed by the rector of St. Mark's to evaluate my performance in the church.

She was in her fifth month of chemotherapy for colon cancer. A tall, stately woman, she appeared to have lost a lot of weight. She told me, "I am 108 pounds dripping wet." Despite the severely debilitating effects of chemotherapy, she carried herself with grandeur. She steadied her walk with a cane in her right hand, but one barely noticed the cane. Her smile was beautiful and constant. She enlivened our committee meetings with quick wit and spirited humor. But I found myself wondering why she bothered to show up for meetings, because her body was so wasted and infected.

We became friends and remained friends during my two years of progression through the ordination exploration process. I drove her to the facilities where her medical oncology treatments were administered. I visited her at her home. We shared healing services and the healing rite at her home. We discussed and often agreed on many insights and perspectives in theological books both of us had read or were reading. She planned our trips from Norfolk to Richmond to hear theologians lecturing at a church, school, or seminary. She regarded her debilitation as an annoyance.

When she was first diagnosed with colon cancer, she had the cancer removed surgically. The surgery alone probably cured her disease. But her oncologist told her that surgery had given her an eighty percent chance of cure; a year of chemotherapy would increase that chance to ninety percent. She was eighty-two years old, yet she opted for chemotherapy. I could not at first understand why she said yes to the debilitating chemotherapy regimen. But then I came to see that she believed in the skill and wisdom of her doctors—to a fault. Despite her chemotherapy-induced incessant diarrhea and fifty-pound weight loss, infected eyes, and abundant mouth sores, Harriet pushed herself onwards, living every moment fully.

Colon cancer wasn't her sole physical affliction. Many years of rheumatoid arthritis had taken its toll. Her cane helped maintain her balance.

Roughly five years before we met, Harriet had dislocated her right shoulder. Physicians were unable to relocate the shoulder into its socket—a typical complication of rheumatoid arthritis. The dislocated shoulder caused Harriet to lose the normal mobility of her right arm and hand.

My first visit to her home brought me face-to-face with numerous watercolor paintings, all created by Harriet and hanging in every room. I was awed and charmed by the beauty of the paintings; I was blown away.

I also noted a marked difference in the style of some of the paintings. Why the difference? Then I realized that most of the paintings had been done with her right hand. The paintings that exhibited a different style were created with her left hand.

Harriet explained that after the surgeons failed to relocate her shoulder, she sank into depression—briefly.

"I resolved," Harriet stated, "that I couldn't remain on the pity pot forever, so I would learn to paint with my left hand"—which she did.

Her left-handed paintings were technically as excellent as her right-handed ones, but their style was more fluid. Harriet thought the left-handed paintings were more spiritual. I am the proud owner of Harriet's left-handed painting of a Christmas cactus.

Ten months into her chemotherapy, Harriet fell, breaking her right hip. Chemotherapy was stopped to allow healing of her hip fracture. What a disappointment! Harriet had planned a trip to Europe upon completion of her chemotherapy. Now the trip had to be postponed for three months. During her hospitalization, while her hip healed, Harriet's body began to heal from the chemotherapy. Her diarrhea stopped. She gained weight. Her multiple infections disappeared.

"I feel one hundred percent better," she announced. "I feel like my old self again! I don't think I need those last two months of chemotherapy."

I totally supported her decision.

Three months later, her hip fracture healed, she returned to her oncologist. He insisted that she finish the course of chemotherapy. Harriet still retained a mistaken, yet deep, faith in the infallibility of physicians. So she relinquished herself to the oncologist's wishes and resumed chemotherapy.

A fatal mistake. The very same day she finished her chemotherapy, she was hospitalized with a life-threatening pericarditis (an inflammation of the sac surrounding the heart, constricting the normal beating of the heart). Pericarditis is a known complication of the chemotherapy she received.

I was at Virginia Theological Seminary in Alexandria. I telephoned Harriet, telling her that I was coming home immediately to visit her.

She sounded cheerful and strong.

"Anne, I've overcome many things in my life. I'm a survivor. This won't get me down. I need to go to Europe."

She dreamed that night that she was packing her bags for a long trip. She would need to get her wedding dress out of storage and have it cleaned for the trip. Because there was going to be a wonderful celebration.

She died the next day.

From inability to let well alone,

from too much zeal for the new and contempt for what is old,

from putting knowledge before wisdom, science before art and
    cleverness before common sense,

from treating patients as cases

and from making the cure of the disease more grievous than the
    endurance of the same,

good Lord deliver us.

    Amen

—Sir Robert Hutchinson[3]

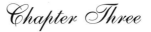

Needing Faith
and Community

My Lord God, I have no idea where I am going. I do not see the road ahead of me. I cannot know for certain where it will end. Nor do I really know myself, and the fact that I think that I am following your will does not mean that I am actually doing so. But I believe that the desire to please you does in fact please you. And I hope I have that desire in all that I am doing. I hope that I will never do anything apart from that desire. And I know that if I do this you will lead me by the right road though I may know nothing about it. Therefore I will trust you always though I may seem to be lost and in the shadow of death. I will not fear, for you are ever with me, and you will never leave me to face my perils alone.

—Thomas Merton[3]

Many published books and articles describe ways to help people cope with disease. Most such publications deal with states of mind of people with disease. People with a positive outlook on life seem to cope better with disease than those with a negative outlook. Norman Vincent Peale's best-selling *The Power of Positive Thinking* was one of the first books written about the benefits that result from a positive state of mind.

Dr. Bernie Siegel, a renowned oncologist, emphasizes the power of love in the healing process. He also has written much about imaging—picturing something destroying one's disease; for example, seagulls chewing at the edges of your cancer until all the cancer is consumed. (Apparently, imaging is easy for extroverts but extremely difficult for introverts.)

Other authors have promoted the benefits of humor in coping with disease.

Jerome Groopman, a famous doctor and researcher specializing in diseases of the blood, cancer, and AIDS and a writer for *The New Yorker* magazine, recently published his third book, *The Anatomy of Hope: How People Prevail in the Face of Illness.*[7] He, too, stresses the critical role of mental attitude when attacked by disease. He attempts to identify a center in the brain that can be called upon to trigger the emotion of hope.

All of these authors, as well as others, teach that there is a definite mind-body connection that helps one cope with disease. I agree—to a point. But I have witnessed many patients deep into a terminal illness where mind-oriented attempts alone have failed. These patients fall into deep depression for many reasons; one being that they believe that they have personally failed because they can't find humor, love, hope, a positive attitude . . . .

That is no way to die.

What is left out of these publications directed to the mind-body connection? The soul. Dr. Bruce Cohen, a professor at Harvard Medical School and director of McLean Hospital, one of the best-known institutions for psychiatric care and research in the United States, discussed with Dr. Groopman the importance of the soul in coping with disease.

"Soul," Dr. Cohen said, "is fundamentally a metaphysical and religious concept, where the divine spark resides. For a person of faith, the soul has permanence, while the body—including brain and mind—does not. The soul is not a product of cerebral chemicals and neuronal circuits." Cohen acknowledged there "is no way to experimentally locate or characterize such a metaphysical entity. It is beyond science; it is a matter of faith. Any physician who believes in the soul should seek to address it in his patients."[7]

A 1995 Gallup poll found that ninety percent of Americans believed in something greater than themselves—God, Allah, Buddha, a higher power, or the One. Eighty percent stated that their faith helped them to cope with disease.[12] Their faith in a higher power is alive through their soul, not their mind.

I believe faith allows for mystery, ambiguity, and doubt. Faith allows one to go forward, not knowing where one is going, not knowing the outcome, and often experiencing pain and suffering along the way.

I believe faith requires extreme bravery and courage.

But I also believe that faith carries the knowledge that God is with you no matter what happens. You are never alone. It is this faith—the knowledge that God is with you—that helps one cope with disease when all else fails.

This same Gallup poll recorded that only forty-three percent of doctors admitted to believing in something greater than themselves. (We learned later that a larger percentage did believe in something greater but were afraid to admit it.) Twenty-five percent indicated they were atheists.[12] (Dr. Larry Dossey asserts that doctors are the most spiritually deprived people on earth.)

The Gallup study was illuminating—and thought-provoking—because it showed that while most Americans relied on their faith to cope with disease, most doctors believed the mind alone is the major coping mechanism.

The Gallup survey triggered a change in medical education: Medical schools began adding spirituality-and-medicine courses into their curricula. (In ancient medical practice, spirituality was the largest component—if not the entire component in the approach to healing.) Doctors, upon hearing of patients' reliance on faith to cope with their diseases, began to look at spirituality in a new light.

In 1999, Dr. Herbert Benson of Harvard University held the first conference entitled "Spirituality and Medicine." Over one thousand doctors and nurses attended the conference. Ninety out of one hundred and twenty medical schools currently include some course on spirituality in their curricula. Psychiatric residencies also incorporate spirituality in their training.

What is the evidence that faith, religion, or belief in the soul influence patients' coping with diseases and medical outcomes? Many studies done in recent years have confirmed that spiritual communities are healthier than secular communities.

My favorite example is a fifteen-year study of twenty-two kibbutzim. Eleven secular kibbutzim and eleven religious kibbutzim were evaluated. Inhabitants of the secular kibbutzim numbered two thousand; the religious kibbutzim contained eighteen hundred.

The reason I like this study more than others is because the demographics in the two groups were the same. The religious practices of one group and the absence of religious practices in the other constituted the one distinguishing difference between them. At the end of fifteen years, the religious kibbutzim had a statistically significant lower number of deaths than the secular kibbutzim. While everyone eventually dies, longevity in the secular kibbutzim was shorter than in the religious kibbutzim.[12]

Other studies reveal that spiritual communities suffer less heart disease and cancer, recover faster from disease, and experience fewer complications from disease than members of nonreligious communities. Life-threatening and terminal diseases are present in all communities. But religious people collectively experience less suffering and experience greater peacefulness than nonreligious people in secular communities.[12]

A spiritual community usually implies a religious community. We know that people can be very spiritual but choose not to attend a religious institution. Sometimes religion is an obstacle to spiritual practice and spiritual growth. Needed now is a study of the well-being and morbidity rates of believers compared with those of nonbelievers. Attendance at a religious institution must not be used as a measure of whether people are believers or nonbelievers. (By the way, all the subjects of the stories in this book are or were deeply spiritual beings, but not necessarily religious. By that I mean some did not or do not attend a house of worship with any regularity. See Chris' story.)

Of course, people living in communities of any kind are healthier than those without a community. Dr. Herbert Benson says that not only do we seem to be "hard-wired for God," but we also appear to be "hard-wired to interact" with each other from infancy on.

I learned in seminary that God lives in community. He lives as God the Father, God the Son, and God the Holy Spirit; there could be no God the Father without God the Son, no God the Son without God the Father, and no God the Holy Spirit without the other two.

We never would have known about Jesus or Mohammed but for the communities of which they were members. How could we know about their lives and their teachings without the communities they lived in telling us about them?

We are meant to live in community—in communion with. Questions of euthanasia and assisted suicide rarely come up among people living in loving communities, and these questions are even rarer in spiritual communities. Such issues are usually raised by individuals suffering alone, without a loving community. Patients cared for by hospice never ask for assistance in ending their lives, because loving support is always present even until—as the poet E. E. Cummings said of his late mother—the beginning.

Anne: How Cancer Changed My Life, Part One
Proof That Lack of Community Can Compound Disease

I was fifty-five years old. I had just taken a job as chair of the radiology department at Eastern Virginia Medical School in Norfolk. I was to assume the position on September 1, 1993. I was taking care of everything I could think of in Washington, D.C., before leaving for Norfolk, so I would be ready to apply my undivided attention to my new duties on day one.

The day before I left D.C., as part of my taking care of everything, I had my annual mammogram four months early. I had absolute confidence in the expertise of my mammographer in D.C. I had no knowledge of the credentials of the mammographers in Norfolk.

When the mammogram was complete, my doctor said she needed some more x-rays—some taken with magnification.

I knew I was in trouble. The doctor spent a long time by herself before calling me in to her office to tell me I had cancer. The lesion was the size of a pea, with tentacles very deep into the upper inner portion of the left breast. I knew her diagnosis of cancer was correct, because I had spent several years reading all the mammograms done at another medical institution.

I was doing mammography when Mrs. Nelson Rockefeller and Mrs. Gerald Ford were diagnosed with breast cancer by mammography. Mammography rapidly became the exam of choice for diagnosing or ruling out breast cancer. I had trained with the physician, Dr. Egan, who developed mammography as a diagnostic tool. I also trained with the physician, Dr. Wolff, who developed xero-mammography (a process, invented by Xerox, that uses x-ray beams to produce an image with blue powder on paper). For three years,

I lectured women throughout Virginia and elsewhere about the importance of having yearly mammograms after the age of forty.

So I knew I had cancer, but I found it hard to believe. I had gotten annual mammograms, all of which were negative for cancer, for fifteen years; now within eight months of my previous mammogram, I had developed cancer. I had no predisposing factors for cancer: No one in my family had had breast cancer; I nursed both of my children; I had no evidence of fibrocystic disease of the breast. That I had breast cancer seemed impossible.

But that I had breast cancer was clear. The cancer had to be treated.

Should I go to Norfolk and take up the new challenge awaiting me, yet where I knew no one?

Or should I stay in D.C., where I knew and had worked with many of the best oncology physicians and surgeons in the Washington metropolitan region and where I had many friends to support and comfort me?

I decided to go to Norfolk. If I became uncomfortable with the mammographer who would be working with me, I could quickly retreat to D.C. The lesion in my left breast was so small and so deep, I wondered whether the mammographer in Norfolk could locate it with a needle for the surgeon.

The day after arriving in Norfolk, I immediately took my mammograms to Dr. Nina Fabizewski. After viewing them, she stopped smiling. She turned to me and said, "You know that you have cancer?"

I asked if she could put a needle in it for the surgeon.

"Absolutely!" she said. "Let me show you."

She led me into the ultrasound room and repeatedly demonstrated how precisely she could locate the lesion. She moved the ultrasound probe over my breast several times. When the probe was over a specific spot of my upper inner breast, she would say, "There it is."

I was fascinated that every time the probe was over the lesion, I experienced pinpoint pain. I normally had no pain in my breast and I certainly did not have any palpable abnormality.

Dr. Fabizewski spent a pastoral hour and a half talking with me, despite her very busy schedule. When I left her office, I had been persuaded that I would be in good medical hands in Norfolk—and so I stayed.

We arranged the biopsy for September 15. I was not worried, for I already knew it was cancer. The cancer had been detected very early—I knew I would be a cure. What I worried about most was how I was going to carry out all my duties as chair while I was facing surgery and probable radiation treatments after surgery every day through December. I knew I would lack my normal energy.

When I told others, including my surgeon, that I had cancer, they always responded, "Oh, Anne, you are such a pessimist. You must try to have a little hope."

No one understood that I had expertise in diagnosing cancer, and I resented their ignorance.

I wasn't a pessimist; I was a realist trying to accept the reality that I would be undergoing prolonged treatment of my breast cancer. I stopped sharing the news of my cancer until after the biopsy proved I had it.

Once the biopsy showed cancer and I shared this with people, some said, "Oh, Anne, that's too bad. Maybe you'll have to change your lifestyle." Or, "Maybe you need to eat differently." Or they would say something else that seemed to blame me for having breast cancer.

I found it very strange and hurtful.

Perhaps people meant well. But I again stopped telling others of my newly detected cancer.

I asked physicians for names of good psychotherapists or good pastoral counselors to help me to get through the surgery and its aftermath. Responses to my queries were also strange and disappointing.

"Oh, Anne, you don't need anyone. You're strong enough. You will have no trouble getting through this."

Then I lucked out. I found a priest who said he'd help me—but only temporarily. But, thanks be to God, he helped me over the next five years, as my pastoral counselor and then as my spiritual director.

I cried for two months. My lymph nodes, surgically removed, were all negative. I had known they would be. I had actually resisted having the node dissection because of my God-given intuition that the nodes would be cancer-free. I called all the well-known U.S. cancer institutes, for I had many professional and personal connections throughout the country. But I could find no medical authority who would agree with me that node dissection was unnecessary.

After healing from the surgery, I underwent ten weeks of daily radiation. My doctors arranged for me to be the first patient in the morning, which would allow me to work a full day.

But I didn't feel like working. I was one of those patients who tire from radiation. I also hated every moment of radiation. I would say over and over again to the radiation beam, "Don't you dare invade me."

I was extremely depressed. I felt very much alone, for I had no real community in Norfolk. There had been no time for me to build a supportive community.

Five years later I learned about Lee's Friends, a very active cancer-patient-support organization that occupied a wing of the church I attended. Lee's Friends assigns trained volunteers to be with people who have cancer. Although I was attending this church regularly, no one in the parish, or outside the parish, ever mentioned the organization to me. I would have benefited immensely from Lee's Friends' ministry. I would not have felt so alone and invisible.

Physicians from my radiology group telephoned from time to time to inquire as to when I would be ready to work full-time. I couldn't tell them. I would hang up the phone and cry some more. My disease had become an illness and society had created my sickness.

The radiation treatment lowered my immune system. I got several colds in a row, all accompanied by fevers. I never had a fever before when I had a cold, nor have I had one since that time.

I desperately needed something or someone very radical in my world to move me beyond my illness and sickness.

See chapter 5, part two, for the story of my healing.

No prayer unanswered is,
If He say 'yes', 'tis well,
Or He answer 'wait',
Rest suppliant at his gate.
He never answers 'no',
But that in time,
Some richer fuller gift is thine.

—R. E. Cleeve[3]

Isabel: Living in the Present

Isabel was ninety-two years old when I first met her. She lived on the third floor of the assisted-living area of a retirement home. She suffered from emphysema. At intervals throughout the day, she would place herself on her home oxygen tank. Nevertheless, she climbed the three flights of stairs to her apartment—"to keep myself in shape."

She was a small, thin woman hunched over at the neck and upper-thoracic area. Her teeth were her own, but obviously had received little care as a child. She spoke with great vivacity and, with little urging, sketched for me her life's story.

She was the second oldest of seven children. Her father had died unexpectedly when she was nine. He left no insurance or savings. The family was destitute. Her mother was forced to place her seven children in an orphanage; she found one that promised to keep them together.

Her mother then worked as a servant in a household where she was housed and fed and paid a small wage. The orphanage allowed her to visit her children only once a week.

Several years later Isabel's mother had saved enough money to rent a very small two-room apartment. One room was the bedroom. She hung a sheet down the middle of the room to separate the boys from the girls. The second room was the living and studying area.

Isabel stopped school at age fourteen and got her first job; her mother explained that Isabel had to work to help provide food and shelter for the younger children.

An insurance company hired Isabel. She was quite good with figures. Pleased with her work, the insurance company raised her pay each year. When she was eighteen, the company told her that despite her excellent job performance, its policy forbade awarding her further pay increases. She had "maxed out."

Isabel asked her mother for permission to work at Kodak, where she would start at a lower salary, but had the potential to make a greater one than she earned at the insurance company. Because more children in the family were working by then, her mother agreed.

Isabel hated working at Kodak. Nothing about her job pleased her. But in that workplace she met a young man—another employee— whom she liked. They married within two years.

Her husband had saved some money, and Isabel was free to find a better job. AT&T hired her for a job in sales. She proved to be very good at sales—so good that AT&T sent her around the country to obtain more business.

A traveling *female* salesperson was a rarity in the 1920s and '30s. Isabel's husband was not pleased with her traveling all the time. But she liked the job and the money she earned, so she kept on traveling and selling despite his objections.

They lived in Newark, New Jersey, and basically were very happy together. After she had accumulated enough money for herself, she stopped working. She and her husband then enjoyed traveling together. They also enjoyed the companionship of many close friends.

Isabel was seventy when her husband died of cancer. They had been married fifty years.

Isabel began a new chapter of her life's story. She and her husband had been very close to another couple in Newark. The wife of this other couple had died several years before the death of Isabel's spouse. The widowed husband, Sam, had moved to a retirement home in Virginia to be near his children.

Sam renewed contact with Isabel following her husband's death. The two wrote each other often. Sam encouraged Isabel to join him in the retirement home "because the people are so wonderful to be with."

At age seventy-five, Isabel moved into the independent-living section of Sam's retirement home. She and Sam married two years later. Sam died when Isabel was ninety.

Pointing to pictures of her two husbands, she said, "I had two wonderful and successful marriages. I loved them both."

It was two years after the death of Isabel's second husband that I first met her. She was upbeat and very pleased with her life. She regretted nothing, not even her difficult childhood. She was disgusted only that she took so long to climb the three flights of stairs to her living quarters.

A year later, she was hospitalized with congestive heart failure, a complication of her emphysema. During the entire time she was in the hospital, she fought to get out and return home. She did return home, but she could not climb the stairs anymore. She died at ninety-five, with a smile on her face.

Isabel was a survivor. I believe that one reason she lived so long despite her difficult childhood was that she always lived fully in the present. Perhaps the ordeal of her childhood had taught her to do that.

The past was always the past for Isabel and the future would be as it would be. Isabel's faith was very deep. She never knew where she was going, but she would go there anyway, knowing she was never alone. That's what faith is.

Look to this day, for it is life, the very life of life.
In its brief course lie all the realities and truths of existence.
The joy of growth, the splendour of action, the glory of power.
For yesterday is but a memory and tomorrow is only a vision.
But today well lived makes every yesterday a memory of happiness
and every tomorrow a vision of hope.
Look well, therefore, to this day!

—Sanskrit poem[3]

Marcia: Living in the Mystery With Faith

Marcia is a most amazing woman. Now in her mid-eighties, she is and has been a premiere real estate agent in Washington, D.C. for half a century.

I have known her for the past twenty-five years, and I became her friend about twenty years ago.

At that time I was living at the College of Preachers on the grounds of the Washington National Cathedral. On the Cathedral grounds, I ran into a parishioner from St. Columba's Episcopal Church who told me, "Marcia desperately needs your help. Please call her."

Not knowing what I was calling her about, I telephoned. Marcia answered.

"Anne, I can't believe it, but I have cancer. How can that be when I feel so well? In fact, I have never felt better."

I drove to her house that night to hear her story.

Marcia had scheduled simple eye surgery, which required a pre-op chest x-ray. Following her chest x-ray, some other images were obtained. She handed me the chest x-ray as well as the other images.

I looked at them for her. Her chest x-ray revealed a smooth mass the size of a ping-pong ball right next to the origin of her main left pulmonary artery. A CAT scan, done three days later, confirmed the mass and detected a few very small lesions at the periphery of her lungs.

Her physicians had interpreted the two studies as evidence of "metastatic disease." They then ordered other studies to try to determine the primary site or origin of the metastatic disease. They found none. They would be unable to treat her until a tissue diagnosis had been made.

That Marcia had metastatic disease made no sense to me. Anyone with that many metastases in her lungs from cancer would be very sick. Marcia was as vivacious as ever, if not more so. She reiterated that she felt healthier than ever before. She was on an extremely healthy diet and had taken many steps to relieve the stress in her busy, productive life.

She had not traveled outside the country and she tested negative for tuberculosis or any fungal disease. I also thought that the mass adjacent to her pulmonary artery was too smooth to be cancer.

I took her images with me to consult with several radiologists who specialized in lung disease. They all agreed that the findings were consistent with metastatic disease, but they also agreed that the big mass looked too smooth to be cancer.

We then performed a high-resolution CAT scan on Marcia's chest. The study added little to our knowledge; only that the lesions were free of calcifications, thus helping to exclude a diagnosis of tuberculosis. The big mass, which appeared smooth on her initial chest x-ray, was definitely smooth.

Marcia next had a bronchoscopy. A tube was passed down her trachea into the left main-stem bronchus, in an effort to get a piece of the mass. The procedure was unsuccessful.

Marcia's doctor suggested opening her chest to directly biopsy the mass. I sent her to a physician at Johns Hopkins, who had developed a far less invasive procedure to obtain a biopsy of the mass by passing a specialized skinny needle through the chest wall directly into the mass. But in Marcia's case, the needle extracted fluid only. Again, cellular pathology was not obtained.

The surgeon, eager to open Marcia's chest, was now very angry with her and with me. But Marcia insisted that she didn't want her chest "cracked open" when she felt perfectly well.

Over dinner, Marcia, her family, and I discussed Marcia's options. Marcia could undergo surgery to open her chest and enable her doctors to directly visualize and biopsy her mass to determine what her disease process was. This way, she would have a definitive answer. Or she could live with the mystery of not knowing what her mass and peripheral lesions were.

If she did reject surgery, we could monitor the mass with CAT scans of her chest every three months. We could decide upon treatment options if the mass changed in size or shape, demonstrating aggressive behavior. We could also make different decisions if her health deteriorated.

Marcia chose to live in the mystery of her disease. She had a deep abiding faith that God wanted wellness for her.

Her doctor, angrily, turned Marcia over to me.

"When she dies," he coldly asserted, "her death will be your fault. She is going against sound medical advice."

So we scanned her lungs every three months for a year, then every six months for two years.

The mass and her peripheral lesions did not change. She remained well.

Ten years later, Marcia had to have a chest x-ray before undergoing extensive dental work. At that time she had more lesions than before, but she was still in good health, except for her teeth.

We gave the doctor at Johns Hopkins another try. His attempt this time led him to a very unusual and odd diagnosis. So we called on the Armed Forces Institute of Pathology for help. We sent all of Marcia's studies to the experts at the institute—her chest x-rays, CAT scans, and pathology slides. There was no unanimous opinion among the experts at the AFIP. They, too, recommended opening Marcia's chest to biopsy the mass directly. Again, Marcia chose to live in the mystery.

Three years later—in 2003—Marcia was hospitalized with severe anemia, which required blood transfusions. I told her to be attentive to the hospital radiologist's interpretation of her chest x-ray. My warning was unnecessary. Marcia was on top of that. Her doctors attributed her anemia to severe acid reflux that had caused ulcerations in her distal esophagus.

Today, with medication for her reflux and a strict diet that eliminates alcohol and other acidic foods, Marcia is doing well. Her blood count is checked frequently; there are so signs of anemia.

She is still aggressively selling real estate. She still entertains friends at home and elsewhere. She travels and participates in book clubs. Her deep faith in God is still alive and well. She moves more slowly in her mid-eighties than she did in her sixties, but significantly faster than most of her peers.

Marcia still lives in the mystery of her disease. She has had two decades of a superior-quality life. Perhaps she will die of her mysterious disease, but not much sooner than she normally would die. She promises me a copy of the autopsy report following her demise.

Marcia is an example of how a body can handle a disease—a disease that manifests itself in images produced by medical technology, but not symptomatically. Whatever her disease is, it seems likely to be one for the medical history books.

Marcia is also an example of how one can avoid allowing a disease to become an illness and letting society give her a sickness. She exemplifies the ability to live with the mystery. The rest of us involved with her, professionally or personally or both, yearn for an answer. We wanted that answer twenty years ago. We want it now.

Perhaps the mystery will never be solved.

Meanwhile, Marcia is living life as she always has—to the fullest.

And the rest of us—her spouse, her children, her many friends—marvel at her yet-to-be conquered spirit.

and set me free, Lord,
 free to try new ways of living;
  free to forgive myself and others;
   free to love and laugh and sing;
    free to lay aside my burden of security;
     free to join the battle for justice and peace;
      free to see and listen and wonder again
       at the gracious mystery of things and persons.

—Ted Loder[10]

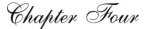

Creating a Healing Relationship: Prayer and Acceptance

A Prayer for Prayer

May we let prayer be.

May we allow it to follow
the infinite patterns of the human heart.
May we learn to practice the most difficult of art,
the art of noninterference.
May we be guided by prayer
instead of attempting to guide prayer.
May we allow prayer to be what it needs to be,
to be what it is.

May we let prayer be.

—Larry Dossey, M.D.[5]

*P*rayer is our relationship with God.

Ann and Barry Ulanov, authors of many theological books, write, "Prayer is the most fundamental, primordial, and important *language* humans speak."—"primary speech."

"Prayer," they explain, "starts without words and often ends without them. It knows its own evasions, its own infinite variety of dodges. It works some of the time in signs and symbols, lurches when it must, leaps when it can, has several kinds of logic at its disposal."[4]

Prayer may be individual or communal, private or public.

Prayer may be offered in words, sighs, gestures, or silence.

Prayer is perceived as a conscious act. But it may also flow from the depths of the unconscious; it may emerge in dreams.

Physician and spiritual leader Dr. Larry Dossey is very important to the healing world today. He was the first physician to lead medical practitioners to recognize the beneficial role that spirituality plays in patients' mental and physical response to disease. He opened the door to allowing discussion of prayer and spirituality to take place between physicians and their patients.

In 1985, when I first started talking about the relevance of patients' spirituality to the practice of medicine, my fellow physicians refused to discuss the topic. I felt as though a door was slammed in my face.

I continued to seek ways to talk about the importance of a patient's faith in his or her response to disease. Not until Dossey's popular book, *Healing Words,*[4] was published in 1993 did the medical profession take its first steps toward respecting the interaction between faith and medical practice.

That physicians had resisted the linkage was understandable. As we discussed in the last chapter, a 1995 Gallup poll determined that only forty-three percent of physicians admitted to a belief in something greater than themselves. More than twenty-five percent declared themselves atheists.[12]

But attitudes began to change. Dossey carried his message to many medical centers, where it was initially received in silence. Then, slowly, a few doctors, and then more, began talking about Dossey's message. Eventually many acknowledged the importance of understanding the role faith played in healing.

The Templeton Foundation was created by the physician Sir John Templeton in 1987. In 1996, it began giving grants to medical schools that incorporated a course on some aspect of spirituality into their curricula. As of 2005, ninety out of one hundred and twenty U.S. medical schools have received monies from this foundation. Medical students may elect to attend such courses. Courses range from the history of the church, world religions, taking the spiritual history of a patient, recognizing the role of faith in wellness, praying with patients when prayer is desired, and many others.

Dossey's interest in the role and effectiveness of prayer began with a little-known study conducted in 1986 and published in 1988 by Dr. Randolph Byrd, a cardiologist in San Francisco. Byrd's study was designed to determine whether and how prayer affected medical outcomes.[4]

Byrd divided into two groups all patients (four hundred) admitted to the coronary care unit (CCU) in San Francisco General Hospital over a period of ten months.

The patients were randomly assigned to two equal groups. A variety of prayer teams throughout the United States were asked to pray for the patients in group one. No prayer teams prayed for the patients in group two.

A prayer team was given first names of patients and told that the patients were in the CCU. The teams were asked to pray each day, but were given no instructions as to how to pray. Each prayer team consisted of five to seven members. Thus, each patient assigned to group one had at least five to seven people praying for him or her each day.

Neither the doctors, nurses, technicians caring for the patients, nor the patients themselves knew to which group the patients had been assigned. Most of the medical teams and the patients were unaware of the study in progress.

The collective recovery experience of the randomly chosen patients for whom prayer teams prayed daily (group one) differed significantly from that of the patients in group two.

Three examples:

- Physicians administered a five-times-greater quantity of antibiotics to group two than they did to group one.
- Twelve patients in group two were placed on respirators. None in group one required a respirator.
- Pulmonary edema (fluid in the lung) occurred three times more often in group two than in group one.

The mortality rate in both groups was the same.

Byrd concluded that prayer positively affected recovery, but not death rate.

His study was flawed. The study's prayer teams were the only control factor. Group two, which was not prayed for by prayer teams, probably was prayed for by members of their families, churches, and friends.

I can't really say what this study tells us; only what it suggests. The best news from the study is that it inspired other studies, which came to fruition through Dossey's work.

Dossey researched medical and spiritual literature and found one hundred other scientifically well-done papers exploring a possible causal link between prayer and health—none published in prominent journals. In the 1980s, the subject of prayer and medicine was not politically correct. The medical publishing world seeks popular subjects.

But research papers found by Dossey reported that prayer lowered blood pressure, hastened the healing of wounds, decreased headaches, shrank the size of tumors, and hastened recovery from anesthesia.[4]

All of the above studies involved human beings who probably prayed for themselves during their afflictions. To remove the effect of self-prayer, the Spindrift Foundation (a publicly supported research foundation dedicated to the scientific research of consciousness and prayer) conducted experiments to document the influence of prayer on nonhuman organisms—bacteria, molds, seeds, plants, and other such things. Prayer affected the growth of all.[4] We know that people who talk to their plants succeed in growing their plants. Talking to plants may be considered a type of prayer.

Dossey reports that prayer's success rate of improving wellness is as great as that of penicillin, without the side effects. I believe that doctors who believe in the power of prayer commit malpractice if they don't pray for or with their patients. I tell patients who are going to surgery to ask their surgeons and anesthesiologists to pray for them. Even if the surgeons or anesthesiologists refuse, the request raises their consciousness—and that's worth doing.

How do we pray? We probably talk more about *how* to pray than we actually pray.

The categories of prayer are numerous: prayers of petition, intercession, confession, lamentation, adoration, invocation, and thanksgiving.

There is ritual prayer, which many denominations engage in every Sunday; conversational prayer, when we talk with God; petitionary prayer, which is specific and goal-oriented; and meditative prayer, when we listen to or feel the presence of God.

Prayer says something incalculably important about who we are in our relationship with God.

Dossey talks about two kinds of prayer.[4] First, directed prayer, which is the more conventional of the two. Directed prayer is guided by instructions laid down by the great religious traditions; it tends to ask for definite outcomes. This kind of prayer is practiced more often by extroverts than introverts.

Dossey calls the second kind of prayer "a state of prayerfulness." It is a state of accepting without being passive, being grateful without giving up. In a state of prayerfulness, one is more willing to live in the mystery, to tolerate ambiguity and the unknown. One honors the rightness of whatever happens. It is a prayer of "Thy will be done." This type of prayer is practiced more by introverts.

There is no wrong or right way to pray as long as one prays with love and intention. For God calls us to care deeply, urgently, wholly, immediately.

Dossey recounts a story about an introverted woman who was diagnosed with colon cancer thirty years ago and given six months to live. Dossey asked what she had done to be cured of her cancer.

"Absolutely nothing," she answered, "except stay in the mystery of it."

Then she added, "Do you think I could get on the Oprah Winfrey show with my story?"

Emily: A Prayer for Peace

Emily married at age thirty-two. She and her husband tried to have children right away, but they had an infertility problem. Results of the usual lab studies were normal, so they proceeded through the series of steps that are initially taken to conceive. The process was an emotional one; the large doses of estrogen given to Emily intensified her emotional ups and downs.

Emily and her husband finally decided on *in vitro* fertilization. The procedure was exhausting. But fertilization and implantation of four eggs started a viable pregnancy of twins.

During the first few months, Emily experienced chronic, severe back and pelvic pain. At twenty weeks, she went to the emergency room with contractions that would not stop. Admitted immediately to the hospital, she was placed on a relatively new medication to stop the contractions. The medicine was injected every four hours through a needle placed just beneath the skin. While the medicine alleviated the intensity of the contractions, it never stopped them entirely. The needle had to be changed every three days. Her husband became quite proficient in replacing the needles.

Emily was allowed bathroom privileges; at all other times, she was to lie in bed. She endured a lot of back pain, for which her physicians could give her nothing, lest the medicine harm her *in utero* babies. Twenty-four weeks into her pregnancy, she was injected with a large dose of cortisone designed to help the twins survive, should they be born too prematurely.

Emily was not a religious person; she attended church on Easter and Christmas and on other rare occasions. But, she had been brought up in a religious family. Emily's mother was a priest and her paternal grandfather was a priest who became a bishop.

Emily's mother, who lived and ministered in a different city, contacted everyone and every church she could think of throughout the United States. She asked everyone to pray that Emily would be at peace throughout her ordeal.

She did not ask for prayers for the birth of viable, healthy children, but only for peace for Emily. Prayers were offered for Emily all over the United States. Emily did not know that her mother had requested these prayers.

Emily told her mother that the hospital chaplain visited her to administer pastoral care. The hospital chaplain was horribly incompetent. The chaplain never asked her how she was doing and didn't even know why she was in the hospital. She didn't even know that Emily was pregnant with twins.

The chaplain did all the talking. She told Emily that if she "would just pray hard enough" her child would be born safely and everything would "be okay."

What a dreadful burden the chaplain placed on an already stressed-out pregnant patient. What if the pregnancy did not have a happy outcome? Were the parents to blame themselves for not praying "hard enough"?

Emily knew much better than that and requested that the chaplain leave the room immediately. Emily's mother remained quiet about the prayer chains she had put in place.

Emily's mother attempted to visit her every other week. About two weeks after the prayer chains began, she again visited her daughter.

Emily greeted her with, "It is really strange, Mom. I can't explain this feeling I have. You know I can lose these twins."

"Yes, I know," her mother replied. (Indeed, the odds were less than one percent that the twins would be born alive.)

"Well, I seem to be at peace with whatever happens," Emily said. "How can that be when I've wanted children for so long and have tried so hard to have them? But I really am at peace with whatever happens."

The power of prayer could not be denied. The prayed-for peace had come.

Emily remained at peace in bed, medicated and monitored for contractions and fetal heartbeats. At thirty-one weeks, her cervix began to dilate and her contractions became even harder. Emily was transferred to the intensive-care unit for maternity patients. The physicians prescribed administration of magnesium sulfate—a fate many considered to be almost worse than death.

High doses of magnesium sulfate are given in an attempt to stop uterine contractions. The side effect of such high doses of this drug is that all the muscles supplied by nerves from the autonomic nervous system become paralyzed. One could essentially lose control of all bodily functions. But within twenty-four hours, Emily was fully dilated and the magnesium sulfate was stopped.

The twins were born by Caesarian section. Each was placed immediately on a respirator. The girl weighed a tad over three pounds and the boy a bit under. They remained in the neonatal intensive care unit for just over six weeks, and were treated for various complications: infection, failure to thrive, and severe esophageal reflux. When they were well enough to go home, they were still attached to heart monitors. The heart monitors remained attached for six months.

Prayers continued.

Five years later, both children are happy, healthy, and unaffected either by their premature birth or by all the medications Emily received during her harrowing pregnancy. The children are extremely intelligent, even for their age. All of their body parts and organs function normally. Emily regained her strength after eleven long weeks in bed. She appears stronger now than ever before. Her miracle babies are now beautiful children.

Medical science and attentive physicians, all gifts from God, figured prominently in the twins' survival in and out of the womb.

So did the determination and dedication of Emily to do whatever she could to assure their survival.

And so did that mysterious peace that surrounded Emily during her many weeks in the hospital—the peace for which so many had prayed.

[O God, we thank you]
　for this mystical, magical moment
　of peace and shimmering power,
　　of grace and prophetic stretch,
　in which you work the miracles
　　of gladdening our hearts yet again,
　　　in spite of painful patches,
　　　　sobering losses, and puzzling trials;
　　of balming our souls with a touch of joy
　　　because we are,
　　　　and are yours,
　　　　　and you are forever;
　　of heeding our prayers beyond our words . . .
　Amen.

—Ted Loder[11]

Sharon: A Prayer for Strength

Sharon was in her late seventies. She stood tall and stately and went about her business as if she had more than twenty years to live.

But she had only a few more years of life. No one could predict whether that few would be one year or four years.

Sharon had myelofibrosis, a disease in which fibrous tissue replaces the bone marrow. She was anemic because she lacked a sufficient supply of red blood cells. She was constantly fighting infections because she lacked a sufficient supply of white blood cells. She was bruising and bleeding because of a shortage of platelets.

But no one spending time with her recognized that Sharon was so ill. She never talked about her disease, except with her physicians.

Sharon had been a career U.S. Army nurse and thus not only possessed extensive knowledge about her disease, but also knew how to take care of herself. She received blood transfusions three times a week at a hospital. She herself carried out a procedure called chelation, to rid herself of the excess iron that accumulated in her body organs from the blood transfusions.

One day when I stopped to visit, she was playing her piano and boisterously singing "Onward, Christian soldiers."

Had she always played the piano? I asked.

"Oh no," she replied. "I just began last year. I had always wanted to play the piano, so I called a piano teacher friend of mine in Baltimore. She could hardly believe what I wanted to do, but she was game. She came down from Baltimore and helped me pick out this piano. And then I started lessons."

"You are a quick learner," I said.

"Well, you know I don't have a lot of time. I go once a week to my teacher, except when I'm too weak to drive. Then she comes to me. I'm having a lot of fun."

We moved through other conversational topics before she told me she had to run to choir practice.

"Choir practice?" I asked in amazement.

"Yes! Since I've learned to play the piano, I have discovered that I can sing. So I now sing alto in our local Presbyterian choir."

"Go to it!" I said with great delight.

During a later visit, she announced that she was preparing for a ten-day cruise to Bermuda with her friends.

"But how can you be away for ten days?" I asked.

"My doctor has been giving me more blood transfusions than I need right now, so I'll be ahead of the game. And I'm taking a store of antibiotics with me."

And off she went to Bermuda. I saw her after her return and was awed by her excitement as she told me of all she had seen and all that she had been able to do. She had had a "glorious trip."

She died six months later.

She was always upbeat when I was with her; she maintained a very stoical attitude and emotion toward her disease. But when I asked at the end of each of my visits if she would like a prayer, her stoicism vanished and Sharon would answer, "Yes, thank you so much." Her words were filled with deep, heartfelt emotion.

Prayer led Sharon to a depth to which she normally didn't go. She often shed tears. I saw them as healing tears.

Prayer freed her to cry, which she usually didn't allow herself to do.

Her stoicism transported her beyond her disease.

So did our prayers.

Onward, Christian soldiers,
marching as to war,
with the cross of Jesus
going on before!
Christ, the royal Master,
leads against the foe;
forward into battle,
see, his banners go.

Onward, Christian soldiers,
marching as to war,
with the cross of Jesus
going on before!

Onward, then, ye people,
join our happy throng;
blend with ours your voices
in the triumph song:
glory, laud and honor,
unto Christ the King;
this through countless ages
we with angels sing.

Onward, Christian soldiers,
marching as to war,
with the cross of Jesus
going on before!

—Hymnal of 1982[8]

Chris: "My Life Is a Prayer"

Chris had just moved from California to a retirement home in Newport News, Virginia. She occupied an apartment in the independent-living section. No one had seen her since her arrival. Meals were being brought to her apartment by the kitchen staff. She did not leave her space for any reason. Her neighbors tried to visit her, but she refused to admit anyone, except her therapists and those who brought her meals from the kitchen.

She apparently had had a stroke that left her slightly incapacitated physically and seriously incapacitated vocally. A physical therapist and a speech therapist were seeing her every day. I was a part-time chaplain at the retirement home. The head chaplain asked me to attempt to visit her. It took me three tries.

The first time I knocked on her door, she opened it an inch and told me in barely intelligible language that she couldn't talk.

Two weeks later she said she was busy with a speech therapist.

Six weeks later, after I knocked again, she asked, from behind the closed door, "Who is it?" I replied that I was the chaplain who had stopped by twice before to see her.

"I busy having lunch," she said.

Could I see her for just five minutes? I wished to find out how she was doing. "Oh, well, come on in," she replied reluctantly and opened the door.

The visit lasted an hour.

Chris was small and thin. She walked without difficulty. Her apartment was immaculate.

She had multiple speech difficulties. She spoke in very short phrases, struggled to pronounce some words, and had difficulty recalling words. Once she had said certain words, she abbreviated them in future phrases. "Catholic" became "K," "Jesus" became "J," and "God" was "gid." She manifested elements of aphasia from her stroke, but some other problem was evident. Not only had she had a stroke, she told me, but also she had had a tumor removed from her larynx.

We sat down and exchanged a few words. Chris became less anxious. I simply listened to her, letting her struggle with her words.

Reassured by my attentiveness, she began to speak more and more. She had a book on a table by the sofa where she sat. The television was on. I did not ask her to turn off the TV, for it seemed important to keep the atmosphere just as it was, so that she would remain comfortable.

Chris explained that she was not going down to dinner or having visitors because her speech embarrassed her. I tried to encourage her to dine with others and welcome visitors. I asserted that people would be willing to listen and wait for her to finish what she had to say, but she just wasn't sure that was true. She had worked very hard with her therapists, but she felt they demanded too much of her. Now she was going at her own pace. Illness (her embarrassment) and sickness (people pushing her to do more) (see chapter 2) were definitely holding her back from interacting with the retirement community.

She picked up the book beside her, telling me that she wished to go to the retirement-home library to choose another. She had been an avid reader before her stroke, but reading the two hundred-page book in her hand had taken her two weeks.

Immediately following her stroke, she could not understand the printed words in books. She was so glad that she could to read again, albeit slowly.

Since the TV was on, I asked if she was able to understand that. She was. She regarded the television as her "lifesaver," for she could see the picture while hearing the words.

But watching TV had a downside. She indicated that an unfortunate consequence was that she had become "hooked on—." I couldn't comprehend the word she was trying to get across to me. She got up from the sofa and went to the kitchen, returning with a bar of soap.

"I hooked on this."

"Oh!"

She was hooked on the daily afternoon soap operas! We laughed together.

Several times during the visit, I let her know that I did not wish to tire her and that I would come back again. To which she replied, "Not yet. Having fun."

Our conversation wandered to religion. She pointed to my collar, "What church?" I told her I was an Episcopal priest. She reported that she was Catholic but she "didn't like the way they"—implying the Catholic Church—"did things around here." Her son's priest had visited her and "tried to get me to go to the K church." He said that if she would come back to the Catholic Church she could "return to God." She told the priest, "Gid is already with me. I don't have to do anything."

I agreed that God was with her, but suggested that she might enjoy attending Mass with her son.

"I'll go when he tells me that he spends more time in prayer than I do," Chris said. "I pray constantly. My life is a prayer. I don't need to go to church to pray."

"I watch the pope on the news," Chris added. "He's a *wonderful* pope! But there is something I don't agree with. Here [implying the geographic region in which she lived], they insist that you must believe in J to get to heaven."

"Who's 'they?'" I asked.

"People here."

"I'm sure that's what your pope would say," I said.

"He not always right," Chris replied. "You know those people who"—she put her hands together in front of her face and bowed her head up and down several times—"three times a day to—?"

"Mecca?"

She nodded yes.

Had she traveled in Arab countries?

She had traveled to many places around the world.

"They are just as believing as we are," she said of the Muslims.

I challenged her. "So you think that heaven is not just for those who believe in Jesus."

"Yes!" she passionately replied. "We are all gid's children!"

I challenged her again. "Even the Hindus and Buddhists?"

"Yes! ALL!"

I told her that I agreed with her, which I did then and do now, and asked, "But how does this fit with your Catholicism?"

"Oh, once a K, always a K," she answered. "But they can't tell me how to believe. Gid is with us all, all the time."

Spiritually, Chris and I were at one. Although her impeded speech limited her oral communication, she nonetheless presented an honest picture of profound belief and unshakable faith. She was such a joy! She had touched me. Clearly, I had much to learn from her and her very deep faith. Imagine one's life as a prayer. What a beautiful life that would be.

Chris was highly animated and totally engaged in our conversation throughout our visit. I admired her courage and perseverance as she struggled to communicate. When she couldn't quite squeeze out a thought, she stuck with it until she bested her vocal obstacle. She never gave up.

And I never pushed her, and seldom tried to express for her the thought or word she struggled to express. I believed that following her stroke, her therapists and her son's priest all pushed her too hard. But now, as she had said, she was progressing at her own pace—she had left her sickness.

That night she went to the dining room for the first time—she left her illness. Though it was difficult for her, she kept going at her own pace. In God's good time, she recovered almost fully from the stroke and laryngeal surgery. She eagerly returned to reading books, which she loved so much.

She died of a major stroke two years later.

She had time to visit with her son occasionally. But she never went to church with him. Her own church was within her being.

The clear bead at the center
changes everything. There are

no edges to my loving now.
You've heard it said there's

a window that opens from one
mind to another, but if there's

no wall, there's no need for
fitting the window, or the latch.

—Rumi[1]

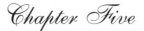

Chapter Five

Giving Life Through Touch

Lay your hands gently upon us,
let their touch render your peace,
let them bring your forgiveness and healing.
Lay your hands, gently lay your hands.

You were sent to free the broken-hearted,
You were sent to give sight to the blind,
You desire to heal all our illness.
Lay your hands, gently lay your hands.

Lord, we come to you through one another.
Lord, we come to you in all our need.
Lord, we come to you seeking wholeness.
Lay your hands, gently lay your hands.

—Rita J. Donovan
St. Bernadette Chapel, Lourdes, France[15]

The most important of the five senses of our body is the sense of touch. The sense of touch is more necessary to us than our other senses: smell, taste, sight, and hearing.

All human activity involves touching. With touch we feel, we love, and we hate. We are touchy. We touch and are touched through the touch corpuscles of our skin.

Let's look at the science of the sense of touch.

Our skin allows us to feel wind, particles, changes in temperature, humidity, pressure, radiation, energy, and light. Our feet withstand the pounding received when we jump, jog, or walk, yet they can feel a light breeze blowing across them.

Our fingertips are one of the most sensitive areas of our bodies. With one tap of our fingertip, we are able to determine whether we are touching paper, fabric, wood, plastic, or steel. Our fingertip can detect a 1/2500-of-an-inch-deep mark etched in a glass. Hairs magnify touch. The tip of a hair one-half-inch-long can feel 1/1000-of-an-ounce of pressure.[2]

We have been given this incredible sense of touch for a reason. Dr. Paul Brand, a famous orthopedic surgeon who specialized in hand surgery and treated a large number of patients with leprosy, suggests that primal listening starts with primal contact through touch. He also believes that, for many of us, love starts with this primal contact of touch.

The power of touch is self-evident. What is the first thing we do when we stub our toes or slam the car door on our fingers? We might say a few expletives. But, as fast as we can, we reflexively cradle the injured toe or finger in our hands. This seems to ease the pain.

Bill, a friend, many years ago broke his tibia (the large bone in the lower leg). His broken leg was placed in a plaster cast that went from above the knee to below the ankle. Bill's toes were exposed.

Bill suffered many complications from this fracture. One day, he telephoned me in tears. Tears were not common to Bill.

"Anne," he said, "I was cooking dinner in a heavy cast-iron pan and dropped the pan onto my exposed toes. My pain is excruciating. My pain is so bad because I can't reach my toes to hold them." Bill was unable to provide the comfort of touch to his own toes.

When small children fall and hurt themselves, what is the first thing they do? They run screaming into the house to be held by their mothers, their fathers, or others who may be around.

Touch is our most trustworthy sense. Children touch objects to make real what they see and hear. When we tell a child not to touch a stove burner because it's hot, the child hears us and sees the red coils; but not until the child touches the hot burner does he truly understand the meaning of what he heard and saw. Though a parent may think that the child's touching the hot burner is an act of defiance or disobedience, it is not. Touching the burner made real what the parent said and what the child saw.

New York City's Bellevue Hospital reported years ago that the mortality rate in the nursery for premature babies was thirty-five percent. In an effort to improve the survival rate, the nurses were instructed to regularly hold the prematurely born infants, cradling them in their arms. With this additional touching, the mortality rate dropped to below ten percent.[12]

Dr. Herbert Benson, internist, author, and lecturer, theorizes that we are "hard-wired" to interact with others from infancy onward throughout life. With infants, this "hard-wired" interaction is primarily touch.

Dr. Paul Brand spent his life reconstructing the hands and feet of patients with leprosy. He said that lepers' loss of ability to feel human touch was far more painful to them than the loss of a digit or the isolation they endured when compelled to live apart from the general population.

Brand considered the sense of touch so important that when his first grandchild was born, he didn't hug him—instead he pinched him until he cried.

"I wanted to hear," he said, "that my grandson could feel my touch."

Doctors, when making rounds of their hospital patients, are known to stand at the end of the bed and pontificate on the present status of the patient. Some are now learning to sit down by the patient and touch the patient's arm or hand while talking to him about his condition. This lets the patient know that he is touchable with his disease. Doctors are finding that this touch is very comforting to patients and hastens their recovery. This kind of touch is especially important with people who have had strokes. It helps them to understand that they are touchable, even if they don't feel the touch.

Just recently, dogs are being brought into hospitals—even ICUs—to allow patients to pet them. This has proved to be beneficial to a patient's healing process.

How unfortunate we have reached the point where touching others in ways deemed appropriate in former times now risks misinterpretation. Now touching others—hugging others—may be labeled as inappropriate, harassment, or suggestive sexual behavior. And yet hugs are healing. Society now limits us from acting upon our normal, natural desire to touch. Healing hugs at the end of a counseling or psychotherapy session between two people of the opposite sex are no longer permitted. Any counseling session that takes place between two people of the opposite sex must be done in a room with a window that permits others to see whether inappropriate contact is occurring.

Touching of a child by a teacher at school is considered inappropriate behavior.

Jesus touched the people he cured. He touched the eyes of the blind man; he held the hand of the girl thought to be dead, but who proved to be sleeping; he put his fingers into the ears of the deaf man; and he touched the tongue of the mute.

Jesus also laid his hands on the heads of people he blessed and healed. He instructed his disciples to heal by laying their hands upon those in need.

Laying hands on the head has been associated with imparting the Holy Spirit. St. Augustine wrote, "The laying on of hands is but a prayer over man. It is in fact a prayer and transmission of grace which takes place within the context of a developing relationship in Christ, and within that relationship there is healing."[9]

George Bennett, ordained by the Church of England in 1935, talked about the laying hands on the head as the means by which the flow of the touch of Christ passed throughout the entire body of the supplicant. He insisted that people understand that it was not *his* nor any other healer's touch that healed; it was the touch of Christ.[9]

Roy Lawrence, a recognized authority on Christian healing in the Anglican church, writes, "Christian healing is concerned not so much with cures as with wholeness; with that harmony with God which helps a person to be more of a person than he was before, spiritually, mentally, physically. In a Christian healing service we seek the touch of Christ upon our lives, simply because Christ is infinitely desirable." [9]

Read chapter 6 for more on the healing rite, in which the laying on of human hands is actually the touch of Christ. But read part two of my story (Anne's story) to see how other forms of human touch can be just as healing.

Anne: How Cancer Changed My Life, Part Two
A Compassionate Touch Healed Me

In Part One, I related how my disease—cancer—grew into illness and sickness as I found myself alone in a new town, with well-meaning but misinformed acquaintances belittling my fears and emotions.

Then, out of the blue, my rescue began. My priest wanted to start a healing center in the church. He assembled a group composed of two physicians, two priests, a massage therapist, and an ex-nun who was running her own healing center. The ex-nun confided to me that the massage therapist, Karen, was a uniquely gifted person with whom I should make an appointment. I had never had a massage in my life, and I was too embarrassed to get one.

But at the meetings of this healing group, after the rest of us had expounded on useful concepts about disease and healing, Karen would quietly speak perhaps two sentences so profound about an example of healing that she left us all sitting in stunned silence, pondering the memorable message she had imparted.

This happened at every meeting. We soon turned over leadership of the meetings to Karen. I was so deeply moved by Karen's insights and the gentle way she expressed them that I felt I just might trust her enough to be massaged by her.

I telephoned for an appointment. She had no time available. I gave a sigh of relief. But then she said, "Wait a minute! I don't usually work on Saturday mornings, but if you could come this Saturday morning, I would be glad to give you a massage."

I was trapped.

But then an acquaintance called to invite me to shop with her in Williamsburg on that Saturday. Shopping with another woman in Williamsburg was surely better than a massage. So I said yes to shopping; I would cancel the massage. But before I could cancel, my co-shopper canceled our trip to Williamsburg. So I reluctantly kept the massage appointment.

I do believe that God was working very hard on me at that point. The massage that day turned my life around.

Karen is a psychic. She worked on her clients' souls as she worked on their bodies. Karen's touch, as I experienced it on that day and other days, was the touch of God. It was this touch that started my healing.

Karen's touch and insights lifted my spirit. Karen massaged me once every two weeks until she discontinued providing massages about two years later. But during that time, her touch and insights led me to really know myself—my strengths, my weaknesses, and my God-given power.

Karen guided me to a much deeper place—a much deeper communion with God than I had ever experienced.

She massaged away my illness and my sickness.

She revealed the divine within me.

Karen is now my dearest friend. We share time together whenever we can find time. And if I need refocusing, she helps me refocus beautifully.

Did I learn anything from the experience of having cancer?

Yes—many things.

I had been a workaholic. But now I established boundaries. For the first time, I was able to call the powerful physicians in my radiology group and tell them not to call me; I would call them when I was strong enough to return.

When I did return to work full-time, I returned on my terms, not theirs.

I know that the physicians who recruited me to be radiology chair were greatly disappointed. Nonetheless, I stuck to what I could do, and I did that well. And I actually became a better chair than the recruiters had expected.

My spiritual life developed along new lines. I learned—and became passionate—about healing, reading all I could on the subject. I met, listened to, and conversed with Dr. Larry Dossey, Dr. Andrew Weil, Dr. Herbert Benson, Carolyn Myss, Dan Wakefield, Margaret Guenther, and Huston Smith.

I grew spiritually so rapidly and deeply, that I left medicine long enough—seven years—to become an Episcopal priest. Now I combine the medical and theological disciplines to teach healing of body, mind, and spirit.

So cancer did compel me to change my lifestyle and my life.

But not in the superficial ways that those who responded to my news of cancer had originally suggested. Touch had changed my life deeply.

For the mountains may depart
and the hills be removed,
but my steadfast love shall not
depart from you,
and my covenant of peace shall
not be removed,
says the Lord, who has
compassion on you.

—Isaiah 54:10

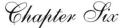

Experiencing God's Touch: The Healing Rite

You are welcome to receive a laying on of hands and a prayer in the name of Christ if you wish to do so for any reason at all. Perhaps you have been ill in some way and have a need for physical healing. Perhaps you are feeling anxious or depressed and have a need for mental healing. Perhaps some temptation is hard to cope with and you are conscious of the need for spiritual healing. Or, if you wish, you may come forward just as an act of commitment, a prayer for spiritual deepening, a symbol of your availability to our Lord. Or perhaps you want to come forward as an act of prayer for someone else, whom you know to be in need of healing. Or perhaps you want to come forward simply because the touch of Christ is desirable for its own sake, quite apart from any by-products it may bring. Whatever your reasons for coming forward, you are welcome.

—Roy Lawrence[9]

he previous chapters on prayer and on touch show that each of these modalities by themselves are extremely important to the process of healing.

In the church's ancient sacrament of the healing rite, prayer and touch are brought together to provide a sacred moment of healing. Perhaps the simplest way to further understanding of this ancient sacrament of healing—the healing rite—is by telling you of my journey from sitting in the pew, not knowing anything about healing, except as a physician understands it, to where I am now as an instrument of healing of the whole being—body, mind, and spirit. Now I am not only a healer, but also I give courses on healing, the healing rite, and how to become a lay healer.

My journey began at St. Columba's Episcopal Church in Washington, D.C., the largest church in the Diocese of Washington. As a regular parishioner, lay reader, and chalicer at St. Columba's, I had observed that while communion was being received at the standing stations, many parishioners approached the altar rail behind the standing stations to kneel before other parishioners or priests standing behind the rail. The parishioners and priests behind the rail were placing their hands on the heads of those kneeling and speaking softly into their ears. My pastoral counselor was one of a dozen or so men and women participating in this laying on of hands. After one Sunday service, I asked her what was happening at the rail. She explained that I was observing the "healing rite"—a ritual that provided another way for parishioners to share their needs and concerns with God and to feel his presence and love.

The following dialogue took place:

"What happens at the rail?"

"A person comes to the rail, kneels, and speaks about a concern to the healer, standing behind the rail. The healer then lays hands on the person's head and prays quietly in the person's ear, bringing the love of God and Jesus Christ into that person's presence."

"What concerns do people bring?"

"Many, many concerns, and too diverse to tell you now. Look at this *Welcome* (quoted at the beginning of this chapter). One may also come to the rail in thanksgiving or for a blessing. One may bring anything that one wishes to share with God."

"What if you have nothing to say?"

"That's okay, too. Many people come forward without speaking a word."

"Who are these healers? Are they special?"

"No. Anyone can be a healer. The healer is not important in this rite except as a channel for God's love. The healer puts his or her ego totally aside, becoming a conduit for God's energy to flow through to the one being healed.

"All healers have to be committed to the ministry of healing. Healers are required to maintain complete confidentiality about what occurs at the rail, not even telling the priest about a troublesome request; they must believe that troublesome requests are conveyed directly to God through the healing rite. The healers also are trained never to talk or ask about the encounter with anyone who comes for healing. But if those who come for healing initiate a discussion about their time at the healing rail, the healer is free to respond.

"Both lay people and clergy are healers, so those coming for healing understand that they are communicating with God, not with the healers.

"Confidentiality is the most essential element of the healing ministry; those who come for healing must understand that they are communicating with God and God alone.

"Healers trust God's work implicitly. If someone at the healing rail reveals that he or she is considering suicide, that concern goes straight to God and no one else.

"Healers are not fixers; they are vessels of God's grace."

* * *

I thanked my pastoral counselor for answering my questions and for sharing so much information with me. I believed that she had really helped me to understand the healing rite. Nevertheless, I abstained from participating in the healing rite for the next two Sundays, although I closely observed it from my pew. On the third Sunday I mustered the courage to go forward. Why did I need courage? I thought that by going to the rail I would expose my vulnerability. Also, I did not know what I would feel or what I would say at the rail.

But I had long watched highly placed officials in our federal government going for healing. They waited in line, just like everyone else. So why couldn't I do the same?

I went forward with my knees shaking. Kneeling at the rail, I said nothing. My tongue stuck to the roof of my mouth. I heard nothing. I felt nothing. All I could think about was my great desire to return to my pew—and become invisible.

Was everyone watching me?

Absolutely not! They were either receiving communion, praying, or waiting in the healing line.

So I persisted in going for healing over the next few Sundays.

My knees stopped shaking.

I eventually was able to pray to God for my own spiritual growth.

And slowly I began to feel a peace from God's touch and prayer.

But I had another lesson to learn, for I chose my healers carefully. I wouldn't go to just anyone. I avoided kneeling before one particular healer who, through my worldly acquaintance with her, I believed to be certifiably crazy. But she was a healer. So I concluded that she must have the necessary commitment to the healing ministry and respect for confidentiality. Besides, if I really believed I was presenting myself to God, it mattered not who the healer was. Understanding that I was presenting my problem to God, I gained the courage to kneel before her for the laying on of hands—and I was transformed. Her touch was infused with incredible energy and her prayer with profound compassion. I was moved to tears.

Thank you, God.

Participating in the healing rite became for me—as it has for countless others—an integral component of the Eucharistic service; a receiving of the "bread of Heaven," "the cup of salvation," and "the touch of Christ."

When I incorporated the healing rite into my corporate worship, I felt more complete at the end of each Sunday service than ever before, and I often sought it out at midweek services.

After departing the nation's capital, I attended Christ and St. Luke's Episcopal Church in Norfolk, Virginia. Christ and St. Luke's offered the healing rite on Wednesdays at noon and at one Sunday service a month. I missed experiencing it regularly. I yearned for its availability at every service. I spoke to the associate rector about it; he likewise wanted to incorporate it into every service.

First, he had to get the rector on board. The rector wanted to be sure that the healing rite didn't degenerate into an evangelistic spectacle featuring the lame throwing down their crutches loudly praising God as they strode away, while others who were lame could not.

The associate rector and I knew that we needed to educate the congregation about the healing rite. We scheduled an eight-week class. We expected about twenty parishioners would show up. We were overwhelmed and gratified when one hundred and twenty appeared. A significant portion of the congregation clearly hungered for healing.

After the class finished, the healing rite was made available at every service, but clergy were the sole healers. I was adamant that lay people be included as healers if we really believed that healing came from God, not priests.

The priests picked me to be the first lay healer, which was *not* on my agenda. Not me. No way. I wasn't a healer. I was the one who needed healing. I wouldn't know what to do. And certainly I was not worthy.

My resistance to becoming a lay healer led directly to the next lesson I needed to learn about healing. The associate rector directed me to review all the beliefs I espoused when I asked that healing be integrated into all of our scheduled services. Did I mean what I taught? If I refused to be a lay healer, he said, then there would be no lay healers. Lesson learned: I had to walk my talk. For three Sundays in a row, I healed with the associate rector. He then cut me loose to be a healing vessel on my own.

Becoming a lay healer further transformed me. Placing aside my own ego came very easily. Listening to so many people in all stages of need and desire was overwhelming and humbling. The only way to deal with the emotions I felt from hearing the petitions of those coming for healing was to turn those needs and desires over to God. I had to trust that God was listening and hearing clearly and that he was providing whatever was needed for each person.

If I thought I had no words to pray, I would wait quietly for a few moments, and healing words would come out of nowhere—or, actually, from God. Prayers flowed through me.

God is present at all times, but his presence is never more intensely felt by me than when I am a conduit for his love and grace. Those coming forward for healing also seem to be acutely aware of his presence. The healing ministry is a transforming ministry.

Some people have asked me about the results of coming to the healing rite. Have I cured anyone of cancer? Have I alleviated depression?

I have no answer for such questions. I do not seek to know about outcomes. And I never ask. Healing is not about results or outcomes; it's about a deepening communion with God.

But I do know that both healers and those who come for healing are deeply moved by the experience. There are people who return repeatedly to the rail because, through the healing rite, they experience the power of the Holy Spirit. The number of parishioners presenting themselves for healing at Christ and St. Luke's grew so rapidly that we had to add more healers for each Sunday.

No crutches were thrown down. But a deeper sense of peace was evident among us all.

I was ordained to the Episcopal priesthood in 2001, after I had already introduced the healing rite to another parish and expanded the healing rite at yet another. Since my ordination, I have introduced or expanded healing in eight more churches.

My passion is to see the healing rite incorporated into the worship service of every Episcopal church in the United States, because it is such a positive, powerful, and uplifting sacrament.

Through this sacrament we know that God is with us, healing us all the time.

Shirley: Healing Hands

I met Shirley four years ago at the request of her chaplain. She was residing in the independent-living section of a retirement home. She had serious heart problems severely limiting her activity.

Shirley was a gracious woman in her late seventies. When I met her, she appeared to be in good health and her apartment was immaculately kept. Despite her healthy appearance, she complained that she was afraid to walk with her fellow residents around the perimeter of the home because of her heart condition.

Shirley had lived in Florida most of her life. About six years ago, while living in Florida, she experienced severe chest pain and was admitted to a hospital through the emergency room.

She immediately underwent cardiac catheterization. Three stents were placed in three coronary arteries. She did well following surgery.

She moved from Florida to Newport News, Virginia, to be near her son. In Newport News, she again experienced chest pain. A local cardiologist scheduled her for a second cardiac catheterization. During the catheterization, the cardiologist made a grave error; he punctured the base of the aorta, so that blood entered into the pericardium (the sac that surrounds the heart). She bled a full cup into the pericardium, causing her heart to stop beating. Extensive measures were taken to resuscitate her. Two cardiac surgeons were summoned to deal with the emergency. Shirley underwent three hours of surgery. Though the actual catheterization never took place, Shirley was alive.

Shirley was never told about the cardiologist's near-fatal error. She was told only that she had almost died. She continued to see the same cardiologist during her recovery, ignorant of the events that had almost caused her demise.

Shirley's chest pain persisted; the cardiologist could not or would not explain why. Her family and some health-care workers advised her strongly to see a different cardiologist. Because of their prompting, Shirley obtained her own medical record and learned about the error made by the cardiologist and the subsequent operation to repair the damage. Having belatedly gained information about the botched catheterization, Shirley switched cardiologists.

She continued to experience chest pain and exhaustion when she exerted herself. A nuclear-medicine image indicated that she needed another catheterization to assess the degree of openness of the stents and the possible necessity for bypass surgery. Needless to say, Shirley recoiled at the prospect of yet another catheterization attempt. At the time I met her, she was willing to try to live her life in her limited way.

She wouldn't walk with her friends. She wouldn't travel or drive a car. She wouldn't exert herself in any way. She had become a cardiac cripple.

Shirley was a deeply spiritual person. Among her many books were several volumes about the near-death experience. She was troubled that during her own near-death experience, she "fell into a black hole"; there was "no tunnel with light at the end of it." She had none of the feelings or visions she had read about in the near-death-experience books. She wondered whether the black hole meant that she was going to hell.

She questioned why God wouldn't just make her stronger without having to undergo risky medical procedures. What had she done wrong to anger him? But she was certain that God did save her life for a reason, even though she had no clue as to what that reason might be, especially if she was to remain so weak.

She and I discussed all these questions. I assured her that God was with her all the time and although she felt that she had been through hell, she wouldn't be going there. I affirmed that God was not the cause of the life-threatening mistake during her second catheterization; the surgeon was. I also echoed her thought that God had saved her life for a reason.

I affirmed her terror of undergoing another catheterization, since the last one nearly cost her her life. She was not afraid to die, she said, but to die by a mistake didn't seem right.

"You know, I could deal with cancer or diabetes or Parkinson's disease, but it seems so strange to me to have a heart problem. Why a problem with my heart?"

I talked with her about the heart being her lifeline, about the heart actually being the center of her being and the center of her thought, which, unfortunately, is often controlled by the thinking brain. I told her about a book, *The Heart's Code*,[16] that might give her more insight into the largely overlooked importance of the heart as the center of thought.

I suggested that Shirley might have a great deal of anger about the whole situation. Her voice expressed anger, but her words did not. Mostly she was in denial about her anger. At one point she admitted anger and then quickly added, "But what is one to do?"

We could do something, and we did. We took her case to the authorities of the hospital where the cardiologist had made the huge error. Not only had he not reported it to her, but also he had not reported it to his peers. Appropriate disciplinary action followed. When Shirley learned this, some of her hidden anger dissipated.

"What I'm also afraid of is that I'll go out to dinner with friends, have a heart attack, and be rushed to the hospital where that particular cardiologist is the only one who practices there." I responded to her expressed fear by saying that it sounded as if she needed to allow her new cardiologist to perform the necessary catheterization to prevent the possibility that the former cardiologist would.

Would she like a prayer asking God to help her decide what to do? She welcomed the prayer.

Would she also like the laying on of hands to accompany the prayer? Shirley said she didn't know what the laying on of hands was.

I explained that the laying on of hands was another way of communicating with God; that as I prayed, I would place my hands on her head and she could imagine that she was receiving the touch of God. I explained further that placing my hands gently on her head as I prayed would not be to cure her, but to bring her some of God's peace.

She said she would like that.

I placed my hands on her head and prayed for God's wisdom and discernment as Shirley wrestled with the decision she was about to make. When we finished, she appeared dramatically moved. She was in tears, yet beaming.

"I had the most incredible feeling during that time," she said. "There was a warmth that flowed from my head through my body. I have only experienced that once before. It was when my husband was alive and in a crisis situation. I had prayed and that same feeling came. I knew that things would be okay."

Three weeks later Shirley underwent cardiac catheterization without any complication. The catheterization determined that all her stents were open and that surgery was not needed. Her physician prescribed a different medication, which eliminated her shortness of breath, her chest pain, and her exhaustion when exerting herself.

I saw Shirly about a month later. She had just come in from walking the perimeter of the home with her friends. She had been out in her car, making many postponed visits. None of her symptoms recurred. A year later she moved out of the retirement home to her own home in Newport News.

This is not a story of cure through the laying on of hands. This is a story of how prayer and the laying on of hands—or the healing rite—helps to bring wisdom and courage to let God work through another's hands. Shirley still has heart disease. But she is living with, through, and beyond her disease at this time. This is healing.

[Give me] . . . silence to cease the fretful conversations
     of my mind with too little else than itself:
silence to calm my heart to an ease,
     convene my senses to an anchored focus,
          hush my tongue to a chastened hold;
until I discern in the silence
     an answer to that necessary question
          which, for the very life of me,
               it has not yet occurred to me to ask;
until I am stretched alive
     and deep to its dimensions,
          and catch, at last and ready,
               your assuring wink at me.

—Ted Loder[11]

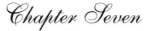

Chapter Seven

Moving Beyond Chaos: Creating Sacred Space

Dear God,
We bring to you those we live with in this society
    but less closely than we would
        were we not so fearfully suspicious
           or so insistent on measuring them
               by our comfortable biases and certainties.
O God, by your mercy, heal the wounds
    we have inflicted on others and ourselves.
Let that healing begin with us
    in the knowledge that with mercy
        comes the power and pressure to risk
           the honesty and humility that will move us
               toward wholeness within each and among all
    through reclaiming and rejoicing in our common humanity,
    as your still beloved family.
                    Amen.

—Ted Loder[11]

I have shared many examples of individual healing. But can healing occur on a global level? Today I feel that I am living in chaos, more so than at any other period of my life. Chaos seems to be present in every domain of our world.

Born in 1938, I was alive during World War II, but was not deeply affected by it. I was aware that certain foods were rationed. My father purchased a motorcycle to "save on gas." I used to ride on the front of the big sheepskin seat of the motorcycle to our victory garden. I loved those rides, but I hated pulling weeds, which was my job in the victory garden. But being very young and quite safe in the United States, I did not experience the chaos throughout much of the world.

I was little aware of the Korean War, for I was in my teens, singing, playing basketball, studying. I was very unaware of tumultuous times in the Sixties because of my studying.

In medical school, we all went to classes and studied for twenty hours out of every twenty-four. One incident that interrupted our study was the Cuban Missile Crisis. A well-loved classmate, fearing nuclear devastation, committed suicide. He left a note telling us that he could not face life in a post-nuclear-war-devastated world. Though shocked and saddened, the crisis passed and our class quickly moved on beyond his suicide.

We mourned the November 22, 1963 assassination of President Kennedy over the weekend and then went back to work. Again, I did not feel the chaos I am feeling now.

I was involved with the Vietnam War. My first husband and I were both physicians. He was a U.S. Army orthopedic surgeon and I was a general practitioner at installations where he was posted. The first year, at Fort Ord in California, my husband saw the horrible wounds of war. The only chaos we felt was fear: "When would my husband be sent to Vietnam?" He never was sent there. He was dispatched to Puerto Rico, taking us far away from even the chaos that existed in the United States because of the American military intervention in Vietnam.

But *today* I feel overall chaos.

This feeling of chaos seemed to start with 9/11.

On September 11, 2001, foreign terrorists guided two commercial airliners into the World Trade Center's twin towers, flew a third airliner into a portion of the Pentagon, and attempted to guide a fourth into another target in Washington, D.C. These atrocities claimed more than three thousand lives, injured hundreds of others, and disrupted families of the killed and injured. The heart and soul of our nation were forever changed. Terrorists are striking around the world. We now live in the shadow of terrorism. And terrorists find no value in human life.

We fight back in Afghanistan, but, at this writing, we still haven't captured the instigator of the 9/11 attacks, Osama bin Laden.

Who isn't aware of our preemptive war against Iraq, in the name of fighting terrorists? Through this war we seem to have collected many of the terrorists into one place. Chaos reigns in Iraq.

Then there is the impasse between Israel and Palestine. Although the two parties are exploring peaceful coexistence, each side desires the nonexistence of the other.

We seem to have no friends around the world—our old friends disregard us.

We have found that a shocking number of prestigious, giant U.S. corporations, stock brokerages, mutual funds, accounting organizations, and banking institutions routinely engaged in corrupt practices that financially ruined millions of workers and their families, investors, and consumers. WorldCom, Enron, Tyco, Arthur D. Anderson, and Marsh & McLennan are among those thus far discovered.

Though the economy is good, good jobs continue to disappear and we are outsourcing manufacturing jobs, the interpretation of radiological images, paralegal work, the handling of insurance forms, repair work on G.E. products, airline reservations, et cetera to India, China, and other low-wage countries.

Our medical care is the best in the world and yet the worst in the world. We've developed our medical technology to such a degree that physicians often don't use their God-given brains and intuition to do right by patients.

The Catholic Church has been decimated by its own pedophilia scandal. The Religious Right is looking toward the end of the world. Homophobia and antiabortion rights elected the last president. The president was said to have been elected on moral issues. What happened to taking care of the poor and the sick?

For me, chaos reigns.

What can be done about it? If we do not occupy powerful positions in government or the private sector—and even if we do—we still must find a way of living with each other and in community in a more loving way, a way in which love transcends feelings of irritation, competition, envy, and resentment towards each other. Such a way would help to resolve differences and further mutual understanding.

Perhaps we can do this by engaging each other in *sacred space*.

What is sacred space? Ann Ulanov, a professor of religion and psychiatry at Union Theological Seminary, exquisitely defines sacred space in a book she has written.[17] As a Jungian analyst, she was invited to address the Norfolk Jungian Society about three years ago. It was here that I first learned of her concept of sacred space and her belief in its absolute necessity.

Sacred space is created when two or more people come together in conversation—either political or personal—and leave an open, yet safe, space for their ideas to be placed and shared. (One might imagine a table in the middle of the conversation on which the various ideas are placed.) Each individual respects the others and respects the ideas that are placed in that space. The ideas are either left to lie in the space or taken up into the life of another. There is no judgment. There are never words of "you should" or "you must." There is no criticism. There is only "I believe" or "I think."

Too often sacred space is collapsed or violated. Fundamentalism of any kind always collapses that space. Whether it be religious or secular-ideological fundamentalism, there is no openness to different thoughts or ideas. Fundamentalism demands strict adherence to its own dogmas, doctrines, and "truths."

If there is no sacred space or openness, there is no chance for change or growth.

If there is no chance for change or growth, then, as Ulanov has said, "we as a people will self-destruct."

Sacred space—when not totally absent—is practiced minimally in families, households, religious and secular communities, workplaces, and the political arena. Let me cite some examples of collapsed sacred space.

We can all agree on the absence of sacred space between Israel and Palestine. The conflict will never be resolved there unless sacred space is established to constructively address the parties' profound differences.

Let us bring this concept closer to home. It is often difficult to find sacred space in our churches. I led a Lenten-study class at a Norfolk church about three years ago. We were to read and discuss together the book, *The Changing Face of God.* The book contained the texts of five lectures given at the Washington National Cathedral by a spectrum of recognized spiritual and theological scholars. All were seeking new ways of being in relationship with God. All were challenging the dogmas and doctrines developed in a distant time and culture that don't make sense in our time and culture.

I was "the only show in town," not necessarily because of my subject matter or me, but because the other courses offered during that Lent were "How to be an Episcopalian" and "How to Find Spirituality in Rock Music."

So I had a crowd. Most were seeking new ideas and thoughts. A few were afraid to even think beyond their very comfortable belief systems. To them, dogma and doctrine were truth.

The course lasted five weeks. As each week passed, the fundamentalist minority in the group became louder and louder, speaking more frequently, and then dominating the group with anger. They violated the sacred space.

One young man said, "I don't understand why we are even reading this book." (I resisted the temptation to respond, "I don't know why you are even taking this course.")

"All you have to do," the young man asserted, "is come to church every Sunday, say the Creed, say the Lord's Prayer, grab the wafer handed to you, believe in Jesus Christ, and YOU ARE SAVED!"

"What are you saved from?" I asked. "And who was Jesus Christ?"

He stormed out of the room in disgust. He saw no need to consider unorthodox views. He was afraid. I had no problem with his leaving. But, for the moment, he collapsed the sacred space we had developed. It was not fair to the other people who were there seeking and sharing ideas and hoping to grow and change. We recovered the sacred space and continued, with the seekers sharing openly.

I'm sure you can recognize this collapsing of sacred space in your own households.

My husband is a flaming liberal in the eyes of a die-hard conservative. He had heard me preach a sermon on sacred space. He loved it. He couldn't say enough wonderful things about it.

The very next day, I innocently asked him, "What do you think about drilling for oil in the Alaska National Wildlife Refuge?"

The question hit one of his many hot-button issues. He got very excited with his thoughts, but also very definite. "Only an idiot would think of doing that!"

He shook his finger at me during his passionate, dogmatic response. He left no space either verbally or physically.

When he paused to take a breath, I asked, "Is there any sacred space here?"

He stopped abruptly, then laughed ruefully.

"No," he said, "there certainly isn't. And I apologize."

Then we had an excellent discussion about it from which we both learned a lot.

Sacred space must exist in any healing situation. Pastoral caregivers, and any person providing care to others must provide sacred space for those receiving care if healing is to take place.

Sacred space is hard to maintain. We do not routinely respect sacred space. Any time we approach another with an agenda, it is hard to give the other sacred space. Our minds know what we want. We become closed and unreceptive to hearing other ways our agenda might be carried out.

Using the concept of sacred space with others builds trust and brings about change and growth. Collapsing sacred space creates distrust, fear, and enmity.

Practicing sacred space must begin on the individual-to-individual level, then hopefully spread to the family, then to the community, and eventually to the world. An incredible vision, but we can't continue in the chaos in which we now find ourselves. This chaos threatens all we hold dear, including the possibility of a better world.

As Ulanov says, "We must find sacred space or we as a people will self-destruct."

Mama Swartzentruber: Giving Is Living

Mama Swartzentruber was more of a real mother to me than my own. She, Papa, and their seven children helped me to rear my two children while I worked as a doctor. They all modeled and gave my children and me unconditional love.

I met Mama and Papa Swartzentruber in 1965. At that time I smoked, drank, and worked outside the home; seven years later I divorced my husband. A smoking, drinking, divorced mother employed in the workaday world was alien to their culture. But they loved us anyway.

The Swartzentrubers were Mennonites—believers that the Bible was the literal word of God. My children and I attended a local Episcopal church; we were not fundamentalists—not even close. The Swartzentrubers never tried to convert us; they never talked about religion unless we raised a question. Sometimes we asked questions because we were genuinely interested in their religion and their way of life. Then, and only then, did they express their views and invited us to express ours.

Mama always sang as she cooked, farmed, made beds, or read her Bible. She and other members of her church taught her seven children to sing in four-part harmony. Their church could not afford a musical instrument to accompany their singing; none was necessary. All the church members sang in harmony. They sang so beautifully, I imagined that it was a choir of angels.

Mama often said, "My home is my work for the church." The Swartzentruber home was always open to anyone who came by. Foreign students attending the University of Virginia were invited out on weekends, just to share a good home-cooked meal with the family.

And what splendid meals they were! Mama made the noodles; killed, cleaned, and cooked chickens from the farm; made the gravy; and cooked the peas she had grown in her garden. And she baked "angel" biscuits. She always served angel biscuits, so named because they were so light and flaky.

Mama took in the homeless, the battered, the raped, and the addicted. She gave them love, comfort, and consolation. Her home was a safe space. Many stayed until they got on their feet again.

Mama's children were always bringing home people from different walks of life. Mama and Papa often had to realign their religious beliefs in order to extend loving hospitality. But with each experience they grew. Mama and Papa came to know so many people from so many places that when they took time to travel around the world, they never had to stay in a motel, anywhere.

Mama sustained three unrelated major diseases. She never allowed her diseases to become illnesses or sicknesses. (See chapter 2.)

The first disease was breast cancer. Following an automobile accident, her physicians discovered a malignant lump in one breast. Before her surgeon performed a radical mastectomy (the treatment of choice at that time), I did a mammogram of her other breast. We imaged a second cancer in her other breast. Bilateral radical mastectomies were performed back-to-back on the same day. She recovered from that horrendous surgery and thereafter was breast-cancer free.

Five years later Mama felt a lump in her neck. Her physicians thought that the lump, which was a lymph node, was most likely a site of metastatic breast cancer. The lymph node was surgically removed and the pathology revealed lymphoma. We sent the pathological material to several prestigious institutes to confirm the diagnosis of lymphoma, not breast cancer.

Mama announced, "I am not going through any kind of treatment to cure me of lymphoma. I know the cure is often worse than the disease, so count me out. What life I have left, I want to live it without medical invasion."

I persuaded her to have a CAT scan and a bone-marrow biopsy to determine the extent of her disease, so that if something led her to change her mind, we could quickly do something about it. For example, if one of her kidneys were to shut down from obstruction by a node, we would be able to relieve the obstruction, if she so wanted. The CAT scan and bone-marrow biopsy revealed no evidence of lymphoma. Except in that one surgically removed node, Mama never manifested any evidence of lymphoma anywhere in her body.

About twenty years ago Mama woke up with indigestion. She often had indigestion at night. When she did, she got out of bed and read or cleaned something until it went away. On that night two decades ago she scrubbed the kitchen floor, but to no avail. The chest pain would not go away.

Papa drove her to the University of Virginia Hospital emergency room. The physicians suspected a heart attack and performed the appropriate tests. The tests detected no evidence of heart attack, so the physicians discharged her home. But on the way out Mama collapsed at the front door of the emergency room. She was swiftly admitted to the hospital. Her physicians advised immediate cardiac catheterization.

Mama refused. And she refused again the next day and the next day. The University of Virginia Hospital transferred her to Martha Jefferson Hospital (the local private hospital) until she either got better or agreed to catheterization. She did neither. She told them she wanted to go home to pray about it.

At home Mama discovered she could do nothing without bringing on the pain again. Nothing improved for four days, so neighbors came in for a healing service. They all laid hands on Mama and said individual prayers. When my turn came, I prayed that Mama would realize that God worked through the hands of others; in her case, through the hands of doctors.

The next morning, she called me and her daughter (a coronary-care nurse) to her bedside.

"I have just one question to ask."

"What's that, Mama?"

"Will I get AIDS from this procedure?"

Her daughter and I were astounded that Mama's fear of contracting AIDS from this procedure explained her refusal to undergo cardiac catheterization. It was laughable, but we didn't laugh. We assured Mama that she would not get AIDS.

"Well," she said, "let's get on with it. Take me in today."

"Today" was the Fourth of July. We told her we would take her in the next day. "Why, don't they work on sick people on holidays?" Mama asked.

We reminded her that she had signed out of the last hospital against medical advice. Because she was not now an emergency case, she would have to wait to be admitted on July 5th.

The next day she became an emergency case. Immediate catheterization and heart bypass surgery were performed. With that behind her, Mama shortly resumed her normal life, eating those good chicken eggs and bacon. She continued extending her hospitality to all.

The following year Papa died instantly from a heart attack. Knowing that the farm was too much to handle alone, Mama, with great sadness, left the farm and moved to a retirement home in Indiana. She carried on her work for the church there. She walked about the retirement home, visiting the lonely, comforting the sick, and caring for the needy. She gave and gave again and again.

She lived this way for another fifteen years, until she sustained a major heart attack. She spent several days going in and out of a coma. All her children came to be with her.

Two of her children were somewhat estranged from Mama. They were living in Alaska. Their income was next to nothing. I paid for their round-trip flight so that they could reconcile with their mother. I believe deeply that it is of utmost importance that estranged children and parents have a chance to heal their wounds before death takes that option away. She awakened when they arrived; the three, along with the rest of the family, shared a week of joy, laughter, and reconciliation.

This major heart attack handicapped Mama's physical life severely. Her nurse daughter took Mama home with her for her final days. During my last visit with Mama, she asked what I was doing and listened to my stories. I asked how she was doing.

"I am so ready to go now; I don't understand why God won't take me."

She died about two months later.

She had given so much from her heart throughout her life. Now her heart had worn out. It just had no more to give.

We all miss her.

She was one of a kind.

She was a saint.

Let us now sing the praises of famous men, the Lord
apportioned to them great glory . . . they are honored in their
generations and were the pride of their times. . . . But of
others there is no memory. . . . These also were godly ones,
whose righteous deeds have not been forgotten.

—Ecclesiasticus 44:1-10 (NRSV Apocrypha)

Bibliography

1. Barks, Coleman. *The Soul of Rumi. A New Collection of Ecstatic Poems.* New York: HarperCollins Publisher, Inc., 2001. Reprinted with permisson of HarperCollins.

2. Brand, Paul and Philip Yancey. *Fearfully and Wonderfully Made.* Grand Rapids, MI.: Zondervan Publishing House, 1980.

3. Cassidi, Deborah, ed. *Favourite Prayers.* New York: Continuum, 2000. Reprinted with the permission of The Continuum International Publishing Group.

4. Dossey, Larry. *Healing Words: The Power of Prayer and the Practice of Medicine.* San Francisco: HarperSanFrancisco, 1993.

5. Dossey, Larry. *Prayer is Good Medicine.* San Francisco: HarperSanFrancisco, 1996. Reprinted with permisson of HarperCollins.

6. Geitz, Elisabeth Rankin, Marjorie A. Burke, and Ann Smith, eds. *Women's Uncommon Prayers.* Harrisburg, PA: Morehouse Publishing, 2000.

7. Groopman, Jerome. *The Anatomy of Hope: How People Prevail in the Face of Illness.* New York: Random House, 2004.

8. *Hymnal of 1982.* New York: Church Hymnal Corporation, 1985. © Church Pension Fund.

9. Lawrence, Roy. *Christian Healing Rediscovered. A Guide to Spiritual, Mental, Physical Wholeness.* Westmont, IL: InterVarsity Press, 1980.

10. Loder, Ted. *Guerrillas of Grace: Prayers for the Battle.* Philadelphia: Innisfree Press, 1984. Used by permission of Augsburg Fortress.

11. Loder, Ted. *My Heart in My Mouth: Prayers for Our Lives.* Philadelphia: Innisfree Press, 2000. Used by permission of Augsburg Fortress.

12. Matthews, Dale A. *The Faith Factor: Proof of the Healing Power of Prayer*. New York: Viking Penguin, 1998.

13. *New Zealand Prayer Book, A.* San Francisco: HarperSanFrancisco, 1989.

14. Nuland, Sherwin B. *How We Die*. New York: Vintage Books, 1995.

15. Oman, Maggie, ed. *Prayers for Healing: 365 Blessings, Poems, & Meditations from around the World*. Berkeley, CA: Conari Press, 1997. Excerpted with permission of Conari Press, imprint of Red Wheel/Weiser.

16. Pearsall, Paul P. *The Heart's Code*. New York: Random House, 1999.

17. Ulanov, Ann B. *Finding Space*. Louisville, KY: Westminster John Knox Press, 2001.

18. Young, Allan. "The Anthropologies of Illness and Sickness," *Annual Review of Anthropology*. Vol. 11: October 1982, p. 257–285.

About the Author

As a practicing physician of forty-one years, Anne C. Brower spent six years in general practice and thirty-seven years in radiology, specializing in the diagnosis of bone disease. She has traveled widely in the United States, Canada, and Europe, teaching and consulting in this specialty, and has served as consultant in the medical care of five U.S. presidents.

Dr. Brower ran the medical residency training programs at Georgetown University and George Washington Universities, the Medical College of Virginia, Duke University, and Eastern Virginia Medical School, and became the first female chair of a medical school radiology department in the United States.

Dr. Brower has received many awards for her expertise, including the 1998 Madame Curie Award for the Most Outstanding Woman Radiologist in the United States. Her first book, *Arthritis in Black and White*, first published in 1981 and now heading into its third edition, is considered a "must read" by radiologists and rheumatologists in classrooms and labs across the country and abroad.

In 2001, Dr. Brower became the Reverend Dr. Brower when she was ordained an Episcopal priest. Transforming her knowledge and passion for healing to address not just the body, but the mind and spirit as well, Rev. Brower went on to introduce or expand the ancient sacrament of healing in parishes across Southern Virginia and Washington, D.C., and to teach and facilitate workshops and retreats on healing across the country. In this book, Brower combines her experiences as a physician, priest, and cancer survivor to present a one-of-a-kind insight into the healing of body, mind, and spirit.